MW00441651

China's "Immortality" Herb
By Michael Blumert and Dr. Jialiu Liu

"This book is a well-written, user-friendly presentation of a remarkable herb. Although new to the West, jiaogulan has a history of successful research and use in China. By supporting and enhancing the body's natural processes, the herb provides a buffer against the physical and emotional stresses of our modern day world. With properties ranging from anti-aging to immune enhancing to energizing, jiaogulan is a welcome addition to our medical bag, as this book is to our library."

Hyla Cass, M.D.
Assistant Clinical Professor of Psychiatry,
UCLA School of Medicine
Author: *St. John's Wort: Nature's Blues Buster*
(Avery Publishing, 1998), *Kava: Nature's Answer to Stress,
Anxiety, and Insomnia* (Prima, 1998), and
All About Herbs (Avery, 1999);

"Congratulations...on the production of a concise informative publication about this promising herb for the Western world. The organization of the chapters permits one to quickly find information to one's questions and the illustrations are clear. As an academic person, I found the bibliography most appealing. It allows me to go to the published literature and guide people who ask about this remarkable plant."

Robert Bye, Ph.D.
Director of the Botanical Gardens
Institute of Biology
Universidad Nacional Autonoma de Mexico

"Thank you for sending me your book. It is very good. You have done a wonderful job for Chinese medicine."

"This book gives an informative overview of the adaptogen and antioxidant herb jiaogulan, known as China's "Immortality" Herb. Such literature is necessary and welcome given the increasing interest in herbal products both as "natural food products" and as alternative medical treatments by both the general and scientific/medical communities. This book is more comprehensive than most monographs/pamphlets on specific herbal formulations. The presentation of clinical studies is especially welcome and needed to validate the medical effectiveness and safety of natural products... This book remains an excellent reference for providing an overview of the scientific studies on this important Chinese herb and allows the reader to judge the potential of its medical benefits in a scientific manner."

Jiaogulan

China's "Immortality" Herb

Michael Blumert

and

Dr. Jialiu Liu

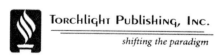

Torchlight Publishing, Inc.

shifting the paradigm

Badger, California

Fourth Printing 2012

Cover design by Stewart Cannon / Ecstatic Creations
Cover and interior illustrations by Carol Blumert
Interior design by Christopher Glenn / Glenn Graphics
Printed in the United States of America

Published simultaneously in the United States of America and Canada by Torchlight Publishing, Inc.

Library of Congress Cataloging-in-Publication Data

    Blumert, Michael, 1948-
      Jiaogulan : China's immortality herb / by Michael Blumert, Jialiu Liu.
      p.   cm.
      Includes biographical references
      ISBN 1-887089-16-0 (pbk.)
      1. Gynostemma pentaphylum—Therapeutic use. I. Liu, Jialiu. 1929- . II. Title.
      R666.G95B58 1999
      615'.32363—dc21   98-51697

Torchlight Publishing, Inc.
For more information, contact the Publisher.
PO Box 52
Badger CA 93603
Email: torchlightpublishing@yahoo.com
www.torchlight.com

Third Printing 2003

Cover design by Stewart Cannon / Ecstatic Creations
Cover and interior illustrations by Carol Blumert
Interior design by Christopher Glenn / Glenn Graphics
Printed in the United States of America

Published simultaneously in the United States of America and Canada by Torchlight Publishing, Inc.

Library of Congress Cataloging-in-Publication Data

    Blumert, Michael, 1948-
      Jiaogulan : China's immortality herb / by Michael Blumert, Jialiu Liu.
      p.   cm.
      Includes biographical references
      ISBN 1-887089-16-0 (pbk.)
      1. Gynostemma pentaphylum—Therapeutic use. I. Liu, Jialiu.
    1929- . II. Title.
      R666.G95B58 1999
      615'.32363—dc21   98-51697

Torchlight Publishing, Inc.
For more information, contact the Publisher.
PO Box 52
Badger CA 93603
Email: torchlight@spiralcomm.net

www.torchlight.com

Preface

Michael Blumert and Dr. Jialiu Liu with this book have brought to public attention another of a group of herbs generally classed as "adaptogens." Adaptogens, as the name implies, are purported to help the organism adapt to stress. Jiaogulan joins such well-known botanicals as the ginsengs, ashwaganda, schisandra, astragalus, glycyrrhiza, and others. This is an important class of agents from herbal medicine in part because conventional medicine has no equivalents to them. They are said to modulate multiple physiological parameters to improve a whole organism response by either increasing or decreasing, as appropriate, different functions where needed. It is perhaps no surprise that drug-oriented researchers have overlooked this class of agents since screening for drug development is usually done in simple cell systems, typically measuring one outcome of interest. Such a screening system may miss significant benefits that require the inter-relationships of body systems to be expressed. Definitive research on adaptogens would need to be in vivo. The numerous health claims made for them have led some to consider them the modern snake oil. Yet, as can be seen in this book, there are numerous studies documenting the effects of the well-known adaptogens. Some far reaching mechanisms have been postulated and some demonstrated—anti-oxidant properties, stress protein modulation, arachadonic acid metabolism, glucose metabolism, etc. This book will help generate continued interest in a group of safe natural agents which may hold an important key to many health problems in modern civilization.

Dr. Carlo Calabrese, N.D., M.P.H.
Co-Director Bastyr University Research Institute

Foreword

I first learned of jiaogulan in the early 1990's when people from around the world sent me copies of promotional literature on this herb and asked my opinion. I checked the journal Abstracts of Chinese Medicine (published in Hong Kong) for medical reports and was pleased to find several studies of the botanical origins, chemical constituents, pharmacological action, and clinical applications of jiaogulan. The findings included in these reports, along with others, are mentioned in this new book by Michael Blumert and Dr. Jialiu Liu. As a result of my investigations, jiaogulan became a part of the clinical treatment programs at our organization's two clinics a few years ago, particularly for the treatment of persons undergoing cancer therapies.

Certain tonic herbs, now called adaptogens, can help protect the body from the stresses of the cancer therapies. Patients who take the adaptogens usually have fewer symptoms of adverse reaction to cancer therapies, they have less suppression of their bone marrow, and, as a result, they have better treatment outcomes (greater tumor shrinkage, longer life, higher rate of cure). Jiaogulan has been recruited to this application.

Adaptogens are also used to normalize blood pressure, blood lipids, blood sugar, and blood oxygen levels; therefore, they are used in cases of hypertension, hyperlipidemia, diabetes, and high altitude reaction (mountain sickness). Further, the adaptogens help the person who consumes them to perform better in sports, in tasks that require mental focus, and in balancing their sense of vitality. In the studies reviewed in this book, these basic properties of adaptogens are shown to exist in jiaogulan.

The Chinese saw the potential for marketing adaptogens worldwide and developed several of their traditional tonic herbs as modern health products, such as wuweizi (Schizandra sinensis),

Table of Contents

Dedicated to
Dr. Tsunematsu Takemoto
and all those committed to the
noble pursuit of
Medicinal Herb Research

Acknowledgments

I would like to thank my publisher, Alister Taylor, for encouraging me to undertake this project and believing in me more than I did myself. Dr. Liu and I would like to thank Mark Blumenthal, director of the American Botanical Council, and Dr. Sidney Sudberg, for reading and critiquing the manuscript; Dr. Carlo Calabrese for reading and and critiquing the manuscript, as well as writing the *Preface;* Dr. Subhuti Dharmanada for his kind and generous offering of so much of his time to read, reread, critique the manuscript and write the *Foreword;* Suzanne Bolte for her editing and creative suggesions; Christopher Glenn for the interior design; and Stewart Cannon and Victoria Ann Taylor for help with the cover design. We would also like to thank Dr. Masahiro Nagai, the scientist who originally discovered jiaogulan's similarity to ginseng, for describing the history of that event to us, and responding very promptly to all our inquiries; and Dr. Shigunebu Arihara, a member of Dr. Tsunematsu Takemoto's research team who extensively studied jiaogulan, for answering our many questions. And finally I would like to thank my wife Carol for bringing jiaogulan to life through her beautiful color artwork on the cover and the pen and ink drawings inside.

Michael Blumert
Los Angeles, California
February 2, 1999

hongjingtian (Rhodiola sp.), lingzhi (Ganoderma lucidum), gouqizi (Lycium sinensis) and dongchongxiacao (Cordyceps sinensis). Jiaogulan turned up quite unexpectedly as a candidate for this group. It had been a relatively obscure folk remedy in China, mainly used for treating lung diseases. It was recently discovered (as described in the current book) to contain the same kind of active constituents as ginseng. In fact, a few of its ingredients were shown to be identical to those found in ginseng.

Ginseng initially became famous because of the root's shape, which is sometimes like a human figure. To be an effective healthcare product, the root has to be grown for many years (6 years is the standard for most cultivated ginseng), which contributes to the rarity and high cost of ginseng. Jiaogulan grows wild over a large region, and provides low cost supplies of the active constituent from its leaves that can be harvested each year. For this reason, jiaogulan is a very appealing ginseng substitute.

Various Chinese clinical trials have shown that jiaogulan is safe and has both chemical constituents and herbal properties comparable to that of ginseng. Proponents of the herb suggest that it might even be superior to ginseng, having a broader range of the active constituents (more variety of saponin glycosides) and producing less of a stimulatory action in persons who are sensitive to ginseng in that way. The body of research supporting the use of jiaogulan is extensive and expanding, so much so that jiaogulan has become a permanent addition to the valuable collection of Chinese herbal tonics used as adaptogens.

Subhuti Dharmananda, Ph.D.,
Portland, Oregon

January 1999

Introduction

The purpose of this book is to bring to light an herb that, although relatively unknown, has been extensively studied in various research institutions during the past fifteen years, and sold in the U.S. for the past six years. There has been a growing interest in this herb, which is not only very similar in characteristics to *Panax ginseng*, but may have some advantages over it. Most of the studies have been conducted in China and Japan, with others in the U.S., Ireland, West Germany, Italy and Czechoslovakia. The findings show that *jiaogulan*, pronounced *jow-goo-lahn*, (botanical name *Gynostemma pentaphyllum*) has extraordinary health-supporting effects on a number of body systems. The results of many research studies are revealed and explained in Chapter Three, both for the layman and the medical practitioner.

"Yes, but a Chinese herb for a Westerner?" This is the reaction I get from many people I meet in my travels. What they don't realize is that pseudoephedrine, an effective component of the Chinese herb Ma huang, has been used for years as the main ingredient in *Sudafed®* and *Actifed®*, a couple of the most well-known decongestants on the market. In addition, Asian ginseng (*Panax ginseng*), which could be considered the epitome of all Chinese herbs, has a variety that is native to North America, called *Panax quinquefolius*, and is known to be a true ginseng, so much so that it has been exported to China and is currently being cultivated there. The herb *Dong Quai* (*Angelica sinensis*) is so widely appreciated in the West for its ameliorating effects on PMS and uterine spasms that we don't even think of it as a Chinese herb. We have all learned that human beings should be judged not by their race or country of origin, but by the content of their character. An herb should be judged in a similar fashion.

What is helping to establish the validity of Chinese herbs, and herbal remedies in general, is the current trend of the natural products companies—to substantiate the claims of effectiveness of a product through scientific testing. This cooperation of traditional disciplines and scientific research can be summed up in the expression *"ancient wisdom/modern science."* Dr. Jialiu Liu, my co-author, heads up one such cooperative team of researchers who have studied jiaogulan. He is a Professor of Pathology at Guiyang Medical College, located in the Guizhou Province in China. Dr. Liu is an active member of many medical associations and has been awarded numerous honors by the Chinese government for his research projects. The College, a Western style Medical and Research institution, has also won many awards from the Chinese government for its achievements in scientific research.

In 1987 the provincial government of Guizhou assigned to Guiyang Medical College a long-term research project: "Studying and utilizing the resources of the natural reserves (specifically the Mt. Fanjing Nature Reserve, a protected rain forest) in Guizhou." A research team of sixteen scientists from various specialties was organized, with Dr. Jialiu Liu appointed as its chief. For many years they studied hundreds of Chinese herbs, then concentrated on jiaogulan, which they found to have many therapeutic and health-giving properties. Eventually, this herb found its way into many prescription treatments at the Guiyang Medical College Hospital, as well as many hospitals throughout China.

In the last few years, jiaogulan has gradually made its way onto the natural products scene in the United States, and is now being sold by many companies, either as a single herb, in teas or in multi-herb formulas. Hence the time has come for an informative book on jiaogulan, from its seed in the ground to your herbal medicine cabinet.

Chapter One

What is Jiaogulan?

Jiaogulan is a plant that grows wild in China as well as many other countries throughout Asia.[1] In China it has been used for many years as a medicinal and energizing tea in the regions where it grows. But, when the scientific/medical community discovered jiaogulan's illness-prevention capabilities as well as its therapeutic qualities, researchers (particularly in China and Japan), began enthusiastically uncovering its great potential. What they discovered was an herb very similar in quality to ginseng, and even in some ways superior.[2,3] They found jiaogulan to function as both an adaptogenic herb[4] and as an antioxidant herb[5] containing many effective saponins named gypenosides, as well as trace minerals, amino acids, proteins, and vitamins.[6]

In China, jiaogulan is sometimes called "Southern Ginseng", since it grows in south central China and because of its similarity to ginseng in chemical composition and function. It is also praised as *xiancao*, "herb of immortality", due to its many health-giving qualities and anti-aging effects. The meaning of the name jiaogulan is "twisting-vine-orchid," being derived from the physical characteristics of the plant.

Jiaogulan the Adaptogen

Jiaogulan is one of the more powerful adaptogenic herbs known.[7] As can be surmised from the word itself, an adaptogen is a substance that helps the body to "adapt" to particular stresses put upon it. The word adaptogen was first coined by

Russian scientist N.V. Lazarev in 1947, and in 1958 was further defined by his student, I.I. Brekhman, to describe a category of herbs that normalize bodily functions. He stated that an adaptogen "must be innocuous and cause minimal side effects in the physiological functions of an organism, it must have a non-specific action of immune enhancement, and has a normalizing action on various bodily functions, irrespective of the direction of the pathological state."[8] An adaptogen is therefore a substance which helps to bring about "homeostasis," the natural equilibrium of the body's internal processes. Jiaogulan has been shown to fulfill quite adequately all these criteria.[9,10,11] According to medical understanding, the action that jiaogulan has on the body is two-fold. One, it directly nourishes the visceral functions (viscera is the general name for all the internal organs) by increasing blood supply to various internal organs, through enhanced cardiac output. And two, it affects the neuro-endocrine regulation to normalize the visceral functions that are adversely affected by various stressors (for example, jiaogulan's adaptogenic effect stabilizes and normalizes the over-irritated brain and sympathetic nerves).

For the sake of analysis, we can divide stress into two types; one being the natural or normal stresses of life in the everyday world, like working hard to get ahead, recreational sports, poor eating habits, anxiety over loved ones, resistance to disease, etc., and the other being the unnatural or overly excessive stresses, like air or toxic chemical pollution, high levels of anxiety, poor personal habits and hygiene, competitive sport to an extreme, the abuse of drugs and alcohol, etc.

These stressors can have a destructive effect on the body. However, the ill effects of day to day normal stresses of life are easily counteracted by the person who leads a relatively balanced life of work, recreation, positive thinking, regular habits of eating and cleanliness, and so on. This person has an immune system that can fight exposure to germs or pathogens, as well as a general resistance strong enough to counteract the normal stresses of life. Exposure to the excessive stressors, however, will gradually weaken a healthy person who does not take care to improve the balance in his/her life, or increase the supply of adaptogenic and anti-oxidant supplements which can help support the body's defenses. Without some form of adaptation to the onslaught of stress, the body's natural equilibrium will be adversely affected, and as a result, illness will likely develop, with the body aging faster than normal.

Adaptogenic herbs actually help our bodies to adapt and thereby counteract the effects of stress. They strengthen the defenses of the immune system, nourish the adrenal glands, and will not deplete the body's valuable reserves of energy, but will bolster them instead.[12]

Dr. Hans Seyle, M.D., a Canadian medical researcher and endocrinologist, after years of studying the effects of stress has concluded that:

"Adaptability is probably the most distinctive characteristic of life. In maintaining the independence and individuality of natural units, none of the great forces of inanimate matter are as successful as that alertness and adaptability to change which we designate as life—and the loss of which is death. Indeed there is perhaps a certain parallelism between the degree of aliveness and the extent of adaptability in every animal—in every man."[13]

Even though psychological adjustment or adaptability to a given situation can ultimately be the solution to many stress-related maladies, the added support given by the adaptogens, both physically and mentally, can help the body to make that adjustment more easily. Not only can adaptogens help the body to withstand and counteract the influence of unnatural or excessive stresses by normalizing the disturbed neuro-endocrine regulation and visceral functions under stressful situations, thus recovering homeostasis, they can also enhance the general health and performance of *healthy* individuals, through their regulating or supporting effects on a wide variety of bodily functions.[14,15]

Aside from jiaogulan, there are numerous examples of adaptogenic herbs, such as Asian ginseng, American ginseng, Siberian ginseng, ashwaganda, astragalus, and schisandra. Although adaptogens generally function in the same way, and have a great many health-giving effects, they are not all the same.[16] What needs to be looked at, in terms of jiaogulan, is the wide variety of therapeutic effects that scientists have demonstrated through their research; i.e., anti-oxidant protection, enhancing cardio-vascular function, blood pressure regulation, cholesterol reduction, positive influence on blood elements, strengthening immunity, etc. which will be discussed in detail in Chapter Three. In other words, getting these benefits by taking jiaogulan could eliminate the need for using a sometimes confusing array of supplements.

Jiaogulan-The "Immortality" Herb

Jiaogulan has been detected by scientific study to have at least eighty-two saponins.[17,18] Saponins are the effective components of jiaogulan and ginseng. (Ginseng has been found to have at least twenty-eight saponins.[19]) These saponins are what accounts for jiaogulan's regulatory effect on many bodily systems, e.g., blood pressure, the reproductive system, the immune system, nervous system, endocrine system, and mental functions. Jiaogulan is highly effective in calming the cerebrum and mental irritations by helping to balance and normalize the brain activity and the sympathetic and parasympathetic nervous systems. As a result, many ailments that are induced by stress might be avoided with its use. Jiaogulan has also been shown to enhance immunity and resistance to disease,[20,21] as well as adaptability to physical and mental stress.[22] Other health-supporting effects of jiaogulan are increased cardiac output, better oxygen utilization, faster recovery from exercise[23] (these effects make jiaogulan the ideal supplement for the high performance athlete as we will discuss later), regulation of cholesterol or lipid metabolism,[24] adjustment and maintenance of the proper balance of stability and excitability of the brain,[25] liver protection (in vitro),[26] improving appetite, etc.[27] Some of these effects are due to the antioxidant action of jiaogulan.

What are Antioxidants?

The key to understanding what antioxidants are is to understand what free radicals are, because the "oxidant" part of antioxidant refers to the oxidation caused by free radicals, in other words, anti-free radicals or anti-oxidation. Antioxidants are substances that disable, or scavenge, free radicals, which are very toxic; they also protect the cell membrane lipids from oxidation by free radicals, through other internal mechanisms. Free radicals are unstable oxygen molecules that are generated in the body as by-products of the natural process of the utilization of food and oxygen by the body for energy (metabolism). They are even more abundantly generated in the body when the unnatural stressors mentioned previously, such as air pollution, pesticides, smoking, etc. are present. The adversely affected oxygen molecule becomes reactive as a result of losing one of its two electrons during metabolism, thus making it incomplete until it can become whole again by "stealing" an electron from a healthy molecule in the body, simultaneously destroying that healthy cell in the process. These destroyed cells then start chain reactions which create more and more free radicals.

These nasty free radicals are the "bad guys" that cause the body to age, just like rust oxidizes (or erodes) metal or air oxidizes (or browns) an apple. The body maintains a natural system of protection against free radicals by producing its own antioxidants, like SOD (superoxide dismutase) and glutathione, two major antioxidants.[28] Under normal circumstances, any deleterious effects would be counteracted by these natural defenses. This would be all well and good, except when the body is overwhelmed by an enormous increase of these unwanted free radicals. This is where the real trouble begins. [29]

Free radicals and the havoc they wreak

Previously we mentioned the excessive stressors that disturb our equilibrium to the point of causing illness. There are many influences that exert a destructive effect on us, such as, stress, industrial pollutants, smog, second-hand smoke, overexposure to sunlight, and more. All these excesses increase the numbers of free radicals, and there is increasing evidence that the oxidative damage to various molecules caused by free radicals may cause such maladies as cancer, atherosclerosis, diabetes, liver disease, inflammation and arthritis, as well as acceleration of the aging process.[30] Under these circumstances we need more antioxidants than the body itself can supply. Fortunately, nature has provided many effective antioxidant sources, one of which is jiaogulan.

Jiaogulan the Antioxidant

There have been numerous research studies that demonstrate jiaogulan's potential as an antioxidant. Experimental and clinical studies have shown that jiaogulan strengthened the antioxidant defenses of the body by inducing synthesis of the antioxidant enzyme superoxide dismutase (SOD) and scavenging free radicals, thus being conducive to the prevention of carcinogenesis, (the production of cancer), prevention and treatment of stroke, heart attack, and various diseases such as atherosclerosis and liver disease.[31,32,33,34,35] Jiaogulan's ability to induce the body's production of SOD is what makes it so valuable in the battle against free radicals. Especially since scientists have noted that SOD when administered orally (exogenously) is disintegrated in the gastrointestinal tract. And even if some SOD molecules were absorbed by the intestinal wall, they would be rejected by the immune system. This apparently would nullify any value in taking an SOD supplement. And the importance of inducing endogenous (naturally produced by the body) SOD, grows more significant as we age. A Guiyang Medical College study showed that with the increase of age there was a proportionate decrease in the production of SOD.[36] Therefore, the stimulation of one's own endogenous SOD is what makes jiaogulan so effective for maintaining good health (and for faster recovery after sports or intense activity)especially as we age.

Demonstrations of the power of antioxidants are being shown time after time in clinical studies, not only with jiaogulan, but with antioxidants such as vitamins A, C, and E; vitamin A precursors, beta-carotene and lycopene; minerals like selenium; and herbs like ginkgo and ginseng.[37]

When taking jiaogulan or other antioxidants to fight against the effects of free radicals, it would certainly be wise to reduce, or avoid the *causes* of excess production of free radicals. Would you continue to add fuel to a fire while you were trying to put it out?

End Notes

1. Flora of China Study, Missouri Botanical Garden, *www.mobot.org*, June 1998.
2. Li, Lin, et al. "Protective effect of gypenosides against oxidative stress in phagocytes, vascular endothelial cells and liver microsomes," *Cancer Biotherapy*. 1993. 8(3): 263-272.
3. Chen, L.F., et al. "Comparison between the effects of gypenosides and gensenosides on cardiac function and hemodynamics in dogs," *Zhongguo Yaolixue Yu Dulixue Zazhi*. Chinese. 1990. 4(1): 17-20.
4. Zhou, P., et al. "The effect of a jiaogulan-danggui compound on abnormal menstruation, premenstrual syndrome and menopausal syndrome," *Journal of Guiyang Medical College*. 1998. 23(1):12.

5. Li, Lin, et al. "Protective effect of gypenosides against oxidative stress in phagocytes, vascular endothelial cells and liver microsomes," *Cancer Biotherapy*, 1993. 8(3): 263-272.

6. Deng, Shilin, et al. "Analysis of amino acids, vitamins, and chemical elements in Gynostemma pentaphyllum (Thunb) Makino, *Hunan Yike Daxue Xuebao*. Chinese. 1994. 19(6), 487-90.

7. Teeguarden, Ron. "Cultivating Essence," *Sante Fe Sun*, Aug. 1996.

8. Wallace, Edward C. "Adaptogenic Herbs: Nature's Solution to Stress," *Nutrition Science News*. May 1998. 3(5): 244, 246, 248, 250.

9. Song, W.M., et al. "Comparison of the adaptogenic effect of jiaogulan and ginseng," *Zhong Cao Yao*. Chinese. 1992. 23(3): 136.

10. Takemoto, Tsunematsu, et al. *Health Before You Know It-Amachazuru*. Eng. Yutaka Nakano Shobo 1984.

11. Wei, Y., et al. "The effect of gypenosides to raise WBC." *Zhong Cao Yao*. Chinese. 1993. 24, 7, 382.

12. Wallace, Edward C. Adaptogenic Herbs: Nature's Solution to Stress. *Nutrition Science News* May 1998; 3(5): 244, 246, 248, 250.

13. Seyle, H. 1978 [1955]. *The Stress of Life*. New York: McGraw-Hill.

14. Liu, Jialiu, et al. "Overall health-strengthening effects of a gypenosides-containing tonic in middle-aged and aged persons." *Journal of Guiyang Medical College*. 1993. 18(3):146.

15. Liu, Jialiu, et al. "Effects of a gypenosides-containing tonic on the serum SOD activity and MDA content in middle-aged and aged persons." *Journal of Guiyang Medical College*. 1994. 19(1):17.

16. Wallace, Edward C. "Adaptogenic Herbs: Nature's Solution to Stress." *Nutrition Science News* May 1998. 3(5): 244, 246, 248, 250.

17. Takemoto, Tsunematsu, et al. "Studies on the Constituents of Cucurbitaceae Plants." *Yakugakuzasshi*. Jpn. 1987. 107(5): 361-366.

18. Liao, D.F., et al. "Effects of gypenosides on mouse splenic lymphocte transformation and DNA polymerase II activity in vitro." *Acta Pharmacologica Sinica*. 1995. 16(4): 322-324.

19. Bergner, Paul. *The Healing Power of Ginseng*. Prima Publishing. 1996. 107.

20. Chen, W.C., et al. "Effects of gypenosides on cellular immunity of gamma-ray-irradiated mice." *Chinese Medical Journal* (English Edition). 1996. 109(2): 143-146.

21. Hou, J., et al. "Effects of Gynostemma pentaphyllum makino on the immunological function of cancer patients." *Journal of Traditional Chinese Medicine* (K9K). 1991. 11(1): 47-52.

22. Zhou, S., et al. "Pharmacological study on the adaptogenic function of jiaogulan and jiaogulan compound." *Zhong Cao Yao*. Chinese. 1990.

21(7): 313.

23. Zhou, Yingna, et al. "Effects of a gypenosides-containing tonic on the pulmonary function in exercise workload." *Journal of Guiyang Medical College.* 1993 .18(4): 261.

24. Yu, C. "Therapeutic effect of a gypenosides tablet on 32 patients with hyperlipaemia." *Hu Bei Zhong Yi Za Zhi.* Chinese. 1993. 15(3): 21.

25. Zhang, Xiaolei, et al. "Effects of a gypenosides containing tonic on the blood lipids in middle-aged and aged persons." *Journal of Guiyang Medical College.* 1994. 19(1):22.

26. Li, Lin, et al. "Protective Effect of Gypenosides Against Oxidative Stress in Phagocytes, Vascular Endothelial Cells and Liver Microsomes." *Cancer Biotherapy.* 1993. 8(3): 263-272.

27. Liu, Jialiu, et al. "Overall health-strengthening effects of a gypenosides-containing tonic in middle-aged and aged persons." *Journal of Guiyang Medical College.* 1993. 18(3):146.

28. Challem, Jack. "Is It Time to Rethink Antioxidants?" *Nutrition Science News.* July 1998. 3(7): 352, 354, 374.

29. Borek, Carmia. "Aging Gracefully with Antioxidants." *Health & Nutrition Breakthroughs.* May 1998: 28-30.

30. Li, Lin, et al. "Protective Effect of Gypenosides Against Oxidative Stress in Phagocytes, Vascular Endothelial Cells and Liver Microsomes." *Cancer Biotherapy.* 1993. 8(3): 263-272.

31. Arichi, Shigeru, et al. "Saponins of Gynostemma pentaphyllum as neoplasm inhibitors." Jpn. *Kokai Tokkyo Koho.* Jpn. 1985. 60(105): 627.

32. Hou, J., et al. "Effects of Gynostemma pentaphyllum makino on the immunological function of cancer patients." *Journal of Traditional Chinese Medicine* (K9K). 1991. 11(1): 47-52.

33. Li, T.H., et al. "Therapeutic effect of jiaogulan on 20 patients with cardio-esophageal carcinoma." *Hebei Zhong Yi.* Chinese. 1992. 14(4): 4.

34. Cheng, Y.F., et al. "Clinical study on the protective effect of jiaogulan oral liquid against liver damage." *Zhejiang Zhong Yi Za Zhi.* Chinese. 1990. 25(6): 247.

35. Duan, J.Y., et al. "Anti-inflammatory and Immune functions of jiaogulan." *Zhong Cheng Yao.* Chinese. 1990. 12(5): 45.

36. Liu, Jialiu, et al. "Overall health-strengthening effects of a gypenosides-containing tonic in middle-aged and aged persons." *Journal of Guiyang Medical College.* 1993. 18(3):146.

37. Borek, Carmia. "Aging Gracefully with Antioxidants." *Health & Nutrition Breakthroughs.* May 1998. 28-30.

Chapter Two

The History of Jiaogulan

Traditional Uses

Although jiaogulan grows in many Asian countries, there does not seem to be any early historical documentation in existence other than in China. The earliest information available on jiaogulan dates back to the beginning of the Ming Dynasty (1368-1644 A.D.), when Zhu Xiao first described the plant and presented a sketch of it in the book *Materia Medica for Famine* in 1406 A.D.. But he recognized it only as a wild crafted plant used as food or a dietary supplement during famine, rather than as a medicinal herb.[1] Later, about 1578 A.D., the renowned herbalist Li Shi-Zhen also described jiaogulan in detail and with a sketch in his classical book *Compendium of Materia Medica*. He pointed out that this herb could be used to treat hematuria, edema and pain of the pharynx, heat and edema of the neck, tumors and trauma. This was the earliest record of jiaogulan's use as a drug, although at this time it was confused with an analogous herb, Wulianmei.[2] However, in the Qing dynasty (1644-1912 A.D.) Wu Qi-Jun in his book, *Textual Investigation of Herbal Plants*, cited the description and sketch from Zhu Xiao's book and added more information about its medicinal usage. He also clearly separated jiaogulan from its confusion with Wulianmei.[3]

Jiaogulan's traditional use has not been widespread in China. It was used as a folk herb in the local areas where it grew wild. Jiaogulan grows mostly in the mountainous regions of southern China, far from the central part of China, an area which has long been known as the "ancient domain of China". This central area of China is where the classical system that we call traditional Chinese medicine (TCM) evolved. For this reason, jiaogulan is not included in the standard pharmacopoeia of the TCM system, and therefore has not had as widespread use as TCM herbs. However, an experienced TCM practitioner in China has analyzed jiaogulan and described its qualities in terms of traditional Chinese medicine, as "sweet, slightly bitter, neutral, warm, enhancing 'Yin' and supporting 'Yang'", and suggested that "it would be used to increase the resistance to infection and for anti-inflammation."

Modern Discovery

Jiaogulan has been used by the people in the mountainous regions of Southern China as an energizing agent. They would take it as a tea before work to increase endurance and strength, and after work to relieve fatigue. It has also been taken for general health and has been recognized as a rejuvenating elixir. People also used it for treating common colds and other infectious diseases. Hence, the local Chinese people called jiaogulan, xiancao the "Immortality Herb," and described it thus: "Like ginseng but better than ginseng." Another story states that in a village near Fanjing Mountain in Guizhou province, the inhabitants would drink jiaogulan tea instead of the more common green tea and as a result many people there were living to 100 years of age.

In 1972 the Research Group of Combined Traditional Chinese-Western Medicine of Qu Jing in Yunnan province did a study on the therapeutic effect of jiaogulan in 537 cases of chronic tracheo-bronchitis. This was the first report of medicinal usage of jiaogulan in modern Chinese medical literature.[4]

Jiaogulan has since been included in the more recent *Dictionary of Chinese Materia Medica*, where it describes the traditional uses for jiaogulan as a medicine. There it is indicated for anti-inflammation, detoxification, cough remedy, as an expectorant and as a chronic bronchitis remedy.[5] Other traditional uses as a medicine have been anecdotally said to be for heart palpitation and for fatigue syndromes.

In Japan, jiaogulan is called *amachazuru*.[6] "Amacha" means "sweet" in Japanese, referring to the sweet component prevalent in the plant, "cha" means tea, and "zuru" means "vine". The name perfectly describes the jiaogulan plant, which grows as a climbing vine and produces a sweet tea from its leaves. Amachazuru has been recognized in Japan since the late 1970s, and its description and uses are included in the *Japanese Colour Encyclopedia of Medicinal Herbs*. Among other things, it is stated there: "Because of the sweet taste of the leaves, it has been used as a mountain vegetable"[7], similar to its use during the Ming Dynasty mentioned previously.

Perhaps one of the more significant revelations about jiaogulan came about in Japan in the mid-1970s. Previously unknown as a medicinal herb, jiaogulan's discovery in Japan came about like many of the world's great discoveries—partially through the hard labor of a dedicated scientist, and partially by accident.

It all started like this: In the 1960s there was a trend amongst some research scientists to find an alternative sweetener to sugar. Although saccharin was in use for many years, they were still pursuing other sugar alternatives. In Japan, the government had prohibited the use of sodium cyclamate, a recently discovered artificial sweetener. Japanese researcher Dr. Masahiro Nagai, presently a professor of Pharmacognosy at Hoshi Pharmaceutical University, recalls:

I had been in the National Institute for Health (NIH) in the U.S. for two years, from 1969 to 1971, when

Dr. Osama Tanaka, a professor in the Dept. of Medicine of Hiroshima University, sent a request to me asking that I send a copy of a thesis on Stevia, which had been a subject of research in the NIH. He was interested in the plant for his study as a safe sweetening agent, which is not a sugar. When I went back to Japan, I decided to study the ingredients of another plant, called amachazuru, for possible use as a sugar alternative which, because of my background in Pharmacognosy, I knew to contain a sweet component.

Upon analyzing the sweet component, he stumbled upon the first discovery by the scientific world of chemical compounds contained in amachazuru that are identical to some of the compounds found in *Panax ginseng*, yet in a completely unrelated plant. He announced his findings at the twenty-third Meeting of the Japanese Society of Pharmacognosy in 1976, at Hiroshima.[8] As it turned out, there was no further investigation of the herb for its sweetness.

At that time, another Japanese scientist, Dr. Tsunematsu Takemoto, whose specialty was herb medicine research, was seeking natural treatments for cancer and other ailments arising from stress, as well as a sugar alternative. His interest of study was in a Chinese fruit, botanical name *Momordica grosvenori*, a melon of the *Cucurbitaceae* (cucumber or gourd) family, known not only for its sweetness, but also for its medicinal uses. His interest in this fruit had been piqued because of its reputation as the "precious fruit of longevity" and as a popular Chinese medicine.[9]

After returning from an unsuccessful trip to Kenya in search of the *Momordica* fruit, he learned of the research being done with amachazuru, an herb in the same family as the fruit he was studying. According to Professor Nagai, "One year after my presentation of the study at the Pharmacognosy Society (1977-78), Prof. Takemoto and his research group saw my reports on the study of amachazuru, and became very interested in studying it." Since the compounds in amachazuru were found to be similar to those in Panax ginseng, and because it was growing wild in the fields and mountains, Dr. Takemoto thought that he had possibly found, in an apparently insignificant perennial weed, an inexpensive and readily available health panacea, right in his native country.[10]

Upon analyzing the amachazuru himself, Dr. Takemoto discovered that it contained four kinds of saponins exactly like those in *Panax ginseng* and seventeen other kinds of saponins very similar to those in *Panax ginseng*.[11] Over the next ten years he and his group of researchers identified and named eighty-two saponins from amachazuru, whereas *Panax ginseng* has been found to have up to 28 saponins.[12] Although these two plants are not related, they contain the same major components: saponins, a substance that has the unique quality of dissolving both in water and oil, and when mixed with water and shaken, will foam up. In *Panax ginseng* the saponins are called ginsenosides, in jiaogulan, or amachazuru, they are called gypenosides. (See Chapter 5 for a more detailed explanation of saponins)

Dr. Takemoto was very excited about this newly discovered herb and he embarked on a mission to gradually uncover all of its potential. Throughout the 1980s, Dr. Takemoto, along with his staff, performed studies which isolated and identified eighty-two saponins, which they simply numbered 1-82.[13] In 1984 they performed three experiments that began to demonstrate amachazuru's many health-supporting and medicinal qualities. They saw that amachazuru increased the activity and strength of mice in a swimming test, showing the herb's ability to improve endurance.[14] Another study on mice showed the herb's effectiveness as a neoplasm or tumor inhibitor,[15] and a third showed the herb's ability (adaptogenic) to prevent the unpleasant side effects of dexamethasone (hormone treatment).[16] These studies used mice as subjects; nevertheless having been tested on mammals, they were a significant marker for the herb's possible effectiveness on humans. This was borne out by subsequent studies on humans. Jiaogulan would prove, in studies, to enhance endurance, inhibit tumors and help protect the cellular immunity in humans, as well as provide many other health-promoting benefits.

Although the Japanese findings were significant, they were only the beginning of the extensive research that would be done on amachazuru. Unfortunately, in 1989 the driving force behind the ground-breaking research, Dr. Takemoto, passed away. As a result, the energy to pursue the research significantly slowed in Japan.

However, interest in jiaogulan by Chinese researchers was growing rapidly, sparked by the results of a nationwide population census taken in the 1970s. The census revealed that, in small regions in the south central portion of China (some villages of Guangxi, Shicuan and other southern provinces), high rates of people per capita were living to 100 years of age. Cancer incidence was extremely low among the inhabitants as well. Scientists from the Chinese Academy of Medical Science in Beijing and other institutions began to research these regions and discovered that the people living there were regularly drinking a tea made from the herb jiaogulan.[17]

Because of the significant results of the census taken in China during the 1970's, and then the boom of scientific interest in jiaogulan (amachazuru) in Japan during the 1980s, many research studies on jiaogulan were undertaken in China, and they have been continuing up to the present. Various pharmacological and therapeutic effects of jiaogulan were investigated and proven by tests on animals and human beings. Tonics and recipes made of jiaogulan have been developed and are being used in Chinese medical institutions. Surveys of the resources of jiaogulan in various portions of China have been made and cultivation techniques investigated. Nearly 300 scientific papers on jiaogulan or its saponins have been published in respected journals, and information about the herb has been formally collected and published in the modern *Dictionary of Chinese Materia Medica*.[18] Jiaogulan has been recognized and accepted by ever-increasing numbers of Chinese people.

From the time of the Qin Dynasty (221 B.C.), the Emperors of ancient China would send various envoys overseas to search for the "elixir of life", but their efforts were always fruitless. Perhaps, the "elixir" has been found by descendants of the Emperors, growing in their own homeland!

End Notes

1. Cheng, J.G., et al. "Investigation of the plant jiaogulan and its analogous herb, Wulianmei." *Zhong Cao Yao*. Chinese. 1990. 21(9): 424.

2. Li Shi-Zhen (Ming dynasty): Ben Chao Gangu Mu (Compendium of Materia Medica) Vol. 2. *People's Health Publisher*. Chinese. 1985. p. 1326.

3. Wu, Qi-Jun. (Qing dynasty). Zi Wu Ming Shi Tu Kau (Textual Investigation of Herbal Plants) Vol. 2, *Shang Wu Publishing House*. Chinese. 1957. p. 559.

4. Qu, Jing and combined research group of Traditional Chinese/Western Medicine, Yunnan. "Study of the therapeutic effects of Chinese herb, jiaogulan in 537 cases of chronic tracheo-bronchitis." *Zhong Chao Yao Tong Xun (Bulletin of Chinese Herbs and Medicines)*. Chinese. 1972. (2): 24.

5. Wu, Y.G., et al. (ed), *Dictionary of Chinese Materia Medica Vol2*, p.1088, Shanghai Science and Technological Publishing House, Shanghai, 1st. ed. Chinese. 1998.

6. Nagai, Masahiro, et al. "Two Glycosides of a Novel Dammarane Alcohol from Gynostemma pentaphyllum." *Chem. Pharm. Bull.* 1981. 29(3): 779-83.

7. Izawa, Kazuo. *Color Encyclopedia of Medicinal Herbs*. Jpn. 1998: 458.

8. Nagai, Masahiro, et al. "Abstracts of Papers." The 23rd *Meeting of the Japanese Society of Pharmacognosy*. Jpn. Nov. 1976: 37.

9. Takemoto, Tsunematsu, et al. *Health Before You Know It.-Amachazuru*. Eng. Yutaka Nakano Shobo 1984.

10. Ibid.

11. Takemoto, Tsunematsu, et al. "Studies of the constituents of Gynostemma pentaphyllum Makino. I. Structures of Gypenosides I-XIV." *Yakugakuzasshi.* Jpn. 1983. 103(2): 173-185.

12. Bergner, Paul. *The Healing Power of Ginseng.* Prima Publishing. 1996. 107.

13. Yoshikawa, K., et al. "Studies on the constituents of Cucurbitaceae plants. XVIII. On the Saponin constituents of Gynostemma pentaphyllum Makino (13)" *Yakugaku Zasshi.* Jpn. 1987. 107: 361-366.

14. Arichi, Shigeru, et al. "Saponins of Gynostemma pentaphyllum as tonics." *Kokai Tokkyo Koho.* Jpn. 1985. 60(105): 626.

15. Arichi, Shigeru, et al. "Saponins of Gynostemma pentaphyllum as neoplasm inhibitors." *Kokai Tokkyo Koho.* Jpn. 1985. 60(105): 627.

16. Arichi, Shigeru, et al. "Prevention of glucocorticoid side effects by saponins of Gynostemma pentaphyllum." *Kokai Tokkyo Koho.* Jpn. 1985. 60(105): 625.

17. Guangxi Ribao (*Guangxi Daily Newspaper*). Chinese. March 4, 1972.

18. Wu, Y.G., et al. (ed), *Dictionary of Chinese materia Medica Vol 2*, p. 1088. Chinese. Shanghai Science and Technological Publishing House, Shanghai, 1st. ed. 1998.

*Note: The authors do not necessarily support the use of animals for testing purposes, but are reporting it here only for completeness, as the testing has already been done.

Chapter Three

Therapeutic Qualities
of Jiaogulan

For more than two thousand years the system of Traditional Chinese medicine has been the primary health
care system in China. However, as a result of the rapid development of Western science and technology which has had such
a great influence internationally, China also developed its share
of Western-style medical universities, if not in quantity, then
certainly in quality. In this age of global communication, tech-
nologies naturally become shared. Today there is at least one
major medical university with its different departments of medicine and its affiliated hospital and clinic in each province,
while other institutions exist in the larger cities of each
province. However, due to the long history of traditional medicine in China, the two disciplines are very often used cooper-
atively.[1,2] Because of the efficient integration of Chinese and
Western medicine, China is on a par with (if not surpassing)
the trend in the West for traditional herbal treatments to be
put under the scrutiny of modern science. Therefore, one can
find listed among the bibliographical databases such as *Chemical Abstracts, Medline, Biosys,* etc., many scientific studies
being carried out on medicinal plant substances in China, in
order to find effective treatments for the various diseases
plaguing modern society, without the harmful side effects of
many pharmaceuticals.[3,4] Such has been the case with jiaogulan.

The methods of testing and developing a drug, or in this case a plant substance, are universal when it comes to scientific or medical research. Testing is the same in the research institutions of China as it is in the U.S. Experiments are conducted in three progressive phases as follows: The first stage is laboratory testing (*In vitro*, meaning *in glass*, referring to the petri dish, vials or test tubes), then animal testing* (*In vivo* or living organism), and finally clinical testing. Their relative importance and as they apply to jiaogulan is explained below:

In Vitro

Laboratory testing is performed using pieces of tissue or cells from an insect, animal or human body cultured in a physiological medium. For example, the direct effects of gypenosides on cancer cells from carcinomas of human liver, lungs, skin and uterus was studied and the results showed that these saponins inhibited the proliferation and growth of cancer cells, indicating that jiaogulan might be used to treat cancer patients.[5,6,7] Although these *in vitro* tests are important for testing the direct effects of jiaogulan on tissue cells, the cells are, after all, isolated from the body and, therefore, these tests are unable to illustrate the real action of the herb in the living organism as a whole.

In Vivo

Animal testing is conducted on living organisms. Some testing is even done on insects, although mammals are the preferred test organism due to their similarities to humans. In the preliminary stages of pharmaceutical development, toxicological tests are first performed in order to test for the possible poisonous effects of a drug, using normal, healthy experimental animals. For example, acute and long-term toxicological tests on jiaogulan were done on mice, rats and other animals. The results of acute toxicological tests (testing within 1 week), showed that jiaogulan/gypenosides were non-toxic to mammals, suggesting that they were non-toxic to humans, with the LD50 (50% lethal dose) of gypenosides in mice and rats being more than 100 times the therapeutic dose recommended for humans.[8] Long-term toxicological tests were done on mice, rats, and other animals (testing with jiaogulan/gypenosides administrated daily over 3 months), showing that jiaogulan and its saponins did not cause damage to any of the internal organs.[9] Chronic testing (over a period of a few years showed that jiaogulan/gypenosides fed to animals was neither mutagenic nor teratogenic, causing neither mutation of the chromosomes or DNA, nor abnormalities of the embryos or newborn of the tested animal, nor carcinogenic (causing no cancer growth in animals feeding on jiaogulan/gypenosides for a certain long-term period).

To test the effect of a drug or plant medicine on a particular disease, testing is performed using experimental animals *with those human diseases.* The experimental testing on animals (mammals in particular) is very important for further indicating the possible efficacy of jiaogulan on the human organism, but animals are, after all, not human beings. The conclusions from animal testing cannot be applied automatically to the situation of the human condition. Therefore, human testing is essential.

Clinical Testing

Clinical testing: After the successful results of testing in the laboratory and then on animals, the therapeutic effects of a drug or plant medicine are studied on humans. Testing is performed using either healthy persons or persons suffering from various diseases, depending on the type of medicine being developed. Until a drug or plant extract is thoroughly tested on humans, any claims of effectiveness of a medicinal herb will be inconclusive.

* * *

Through the above-mentioned three kinds of testing (when available), the effectiveness of jiaogulan will be illustrated below in two different ways. First, a general summary of the scientific studies pertaining to each claimed therapeutic quality for jiaogulan (numbered 1 through 10 below) will be presented. Then, for the practitioner or those with knowledge of medical terminology, a technically detailed explanation of the various experiments, along with their results and conclusions, is given.

Therapeutic Qualities of Jiaogulan

1) Antioxidant
2) Adaptogen
3) Enhancing cardio-vascular function
4) Lowering high blood pressure
5) Lowering cholesterol
6) Preventing heart attack and stroke
7) Strengthening resistance (enhancing white blood cell formation)
8) Strengthening immunity
9) Cancer inhibition
10) Others

Summaries of Research Studies which are the basis for the therapeutic claims of Jiaogulan:

Jiaogulan's Antioxidant Qualities

General Summary

According to a research study at Loma Linda University in California: "There is growing evidence that free radical damage caused by oxidation of cell membrane lipids and biological molecules is closely related to a variety of maladies such as cancer, atherosclerosis, diabetes, ischemic lesions, liver disease, arthritis, inflammation and the regressive changes of the aging process."[10] Accordingly, the antioxidant effect of jiaogulan has attracted much attention of scientists and has been confirmed by many research studies. The results of the laboratory test which follows suggest that the extensive antioxidant effect of gypenosides may be valuable in the prevention and treatment of various diseases such as atherosclerosis, liver disease and inflammation.

Through the testing on animals, scientists found that gypenosides protected the experimental animals from various kinds of oxidative damage which was induced by introduction of free radicals. Also shown was an anti-senility effect of gypenosides and a correlation between the reduction of free radical damage and delaying of the aging process.

Based on the results of clinical testing (human), jiaogulan/gypenosides are used to treat inflammation, ischemia and infarction of the heart and brain (infarction means destruction of tissue cells due to ischemia or lack of blood; infarction of the heart causes heart attack; infarction of the brain causes stroke), and can delay senility and retard the aging process, thus confirming the powerful antioxidant quality of jiaogulan.

Research

Laboratory Experiments: Li Lin, et al. of Loma Linda University studied the antioxidant effect of gypenosides using various models of oxidative stress in phagocytes, liver microsomes and vascular endothelial cells. They found that gypenosides decreased superoxide anions and hydrogen peroxide content in human neutrophils and diminished chemi-luminescent oxidative burst triggered by zymosan in human monocytes and murine macrophages. An increase of lipid peroxidation induced by $Fe2+$/cysteine, ascorbate/NADPh or hydrogen peroxide in liver microsomes and vascular endothelial cells was inhib-ited by gypenosides. It was also found that gypeno-sides protected biomembranes from oxidative injury by reversing the decreased membrane fluidity of liver microsomes and mitochondria, increasing mitochon-drial enzyme activity in vascular endothelial cells and decreasing intracellular lactate dehydrogenase leakage from these cells.[11]

Animal Studies: Dai et al. of Guiyang Medical College found that gypenosides could increase the SOD activ-ity and lower the MDA content of the brain tissue in mice with chronic fluorosis, whose SOD activity of the brain tissue was decreased and the MDA content increased as compared with the normal control mice.[12] Cheng et al. also found that in mice with chronic fluorosis, the depressed SOD activity and increased MDA content of the kidney tissue were improved to the normal range when taking gypeno-sides for three months.[13]

Clinical Testing: A study of 80 patients with endemic fluorosis at Guiyang Medical College found that a 10ml dose of a gypenosides/Danshen (*Salvia miltior-rhiza*) recipe could increase their erythrocite SOD level and lower their serum MDA content. In their study, the patients, aged 42-55, were divided into 3 groups: Group 1-30 patients, 15 male and 15 female, were treated with gypenosides recipe, 10ml twice a day consecutively for 5 months. Group 2-30 patients, 15 male and 15 female, were treated with borax in kiwifruit juice (1g in 10ml), 10ml twice a day for 5 months. Group 3-20 patients, 10 male and 10 female, took kiwifruit juice as a placebo. Twenty other persons of the same age group served as the normal control. The results showed that in the patients with chronic fluorosis, the erythrocyte SOD lowered and serum MDA raised as compared with the normal, healthy persons. After consecutive oral administration of gypenosides/Danshen/Kiwi juice recipe for 5 months, the erythrocyte SOD raised from $847+/-214$ ng/mgHb to $1136+/-203$ ng/mgHg ($P<0.05$); and serum MDA lowered from $0.168+/-0.018$ OD535/0.5ml to $0.136+/-0.023$ OD535/0.5ml ($P<0.05$). The patients showed no significant change in erythrocyte SOD and serum MDA after using Borax/Kiwi juice or Kiwi fruit juice (as a placebo). The results indicated that the gypenoside recipe can increase erythrocyte SOD and decrease serum MDA in patients with chronic endemic fluorosis, where the former was lowered and the latter raised by fluorine intoxication.[14]

Another study of 610 healthy persons, 50-90 years of age, compared the effects of jiaogulan using young persons aged 14-17 years of age as the control. They found that with the increase of age, the serum SOD level decreased and the serum MDA content increased. Oral administration of a gypenosides/Danshen recipe, 10 ml/vial twice a day (each vial containing 20 mg of gypenosides), consecutively for 1 month, increased the SOD level and decreased the MDA content to the normal levels of young persons. The data showed: in the 70-90 year old group, a 21.4% decrease in serum MDA and a 282.8% increase in serum SOD; in the 50-69 year old group, a 15.6% decrease in serum MDA and a 116.1% increase in serum SOD; and in the 14-17 year old (control) group, no significant difference in serum MDA level or SOD level.[15]

In order to clarify the problem of whether the above antioxidant action is due to Danshen or not, the Guiyang Medical College group performed an additional study with Danshen on 20 patients with fluorosis and 20 healthy persons aged 55-70 years old. After taking Danshen extract, 100mg/ml twice a day for one month, the patients and healthy aged persons showed no increase in erythrocyte SOD, although they exhibited a lowered MDA content. The results indicated that Danshen also exerted an antioxidant effect in synergy with the gypenosides, but its antioxidant action was not through the induction of synthesis of SOD.[16]

The results of these two clinical studies showed that gypenosides can induce endogenous production of SOD, which can scavenge free radicals, hence preventing the lipid peroxidation of cell membrane and lowering the production of MDA.

Jiaogulan's Adaptogenic Effects

General Summary

The stress and pressures of modern life which are caused by various strong environmental and psychological stimuli pro-

38

duce stress syndrome, by which the equilibrium between various organs of the body, and the interior stability of the organism as a whole (homeostasis) are disturbed, thus resulting in various diseases such as gastric ulcer, hypertension, neuralgia, psychosis, etc. In order to protect oneself from stress—daily exercise, balanced diet, regular eating and sleeping habits, and a proper balance of work and relaxation—are all important. Still, adaptogens or, as they are sometimes called, tonics have their part to play by helping the body to adapt to the stress and maintain its homeostasis. Jiaogulan/gypenosides have been proven in animal and human testing to be a highly effective adaptogenic tonic.

Chinese scientists found that jiaogulan exerts a bi-phasic action on the central nervous system, calming the nerves when they were irritated and exciting the nerves when they were depressed. Through adjusting the balance of the central nervous system (including the brain, sympathetic and parasympathetic nervous systems) and toning the endocrine system, jiaogulan/gypenosides maintained and normalized the functional equilibrium between the organs of the body and then bolstered the stability of the organism as a whole. Hence jiaogulan has been widely used as an adaptogenic tonic for maintaining normal vital functions and heightening the endurance and resistance to various injurious stimuli.

Research

Animal Studies: Zhou et al. showed the adaptogenic effects of jiaogulan on mice, reporting that gypenosides enhanced the endurance and resistance to hypoxia (lack of oxygen), forced overloaded exercise, electric stimulus, and high temperature.[17] Song carried out a similar study and compared the effects of jiaogulan to ginseng. The results showed that jiaogulan, which functions similarly to ginseng, might be used as an adaptogenic agent.[18]

Clinical Testing: Jiaogulan has been shown to increase the excitability and stability of the brain during athletic competition. The Guiyang Medical College group carried out testing on more than 300 professional athletes, including athletes of the China National Skating Team. All of the tested athletes reported that oral use of a gypenosides/Danshen recipe taken before the competition made them vigorous and alert, with quick reflexes and less nervousness. A control group taking Danshen extract alone did not feel increased stability and excitability of the nervous system during competition, although they also felt increased energy and endurance.[19,20] Jiaogulan/gypenosides showed effectiveness in treating insomnia due to anxiety and irritation when the Guiyang Medical College group studied 112 cases, and showed that gypenosides could improve sleep, with the effectiveness rate being 89-95%.[21]

Jiaogulan's ability to enhance cardiovascular function

General Summary

Jiaogulan improved the efficiency in the pumping action of the heart musculature, so that the heart does not work so hard to produce the same amount of blood flow, as demonstrated in the animal study that follows, where jiaogulan also proved to be more effective than ginseng. The results of human studies confirm that gypenosides can enhance the contractility of the heart muscle and heart pumping function. Based on these findings, gypenosides alone or in combination with other herbs can be used as an energizing tonic for athletes, to produce an enhance-

ment of physical performance, particularly in the area of endurance and recovery.

Research

Animal Studies: Research has shown that jiaogulan exerted a favorable effect on the heart and blood vessels. Chen et al. of the Hunan Academy of Traditional Chinese medicine and Materia Medica investigated the effects of gypenosides on the heart function and hemodynamics in anesthetized open-chest dogs, and found that gypenosides, 5-10mg/kg i.v., significantly lowered systolic pressure, diastolic pressure and mean arterial pressure, and markedly decreased total peripheral vessel resistance, brain vessel resistance, and coronary resistance. The coronary flow was raised and the heart rate lowered by gypenosides. The lowering of myocardial oxygen consumption after the administration of gypenosides could be explained by the decreasing of the cardiac tension-time index and the slowing of the heart rate. Nevertheless, it was significant that gypenosides affected the myocardial contractility and heart pump function. In this study a comparison of the effectiveness was made between jiaogulan/gypenosides and ginsenosides from *Panax ginseng*. Gypenosides were shown to be more potent.[22]

Clinical Testing: The Guiyang Medical College group also confirmed the same effect on human beings as in the animal study above. They carried out tests in 30 normal healthy persons and 220 athletes, using color DOPLER examination. They found that 30 minutes after oral administration of a single dose of gypenosides combined with other Chinese medicinal herbs,

100% of the tested subjects reacted positively; the stroke volume and cardiac output increased; the left ventricular end-systolic diameter decreased and the left ventricular end-diastolic diameter increased, while the heart rate and arterial blood pressure did not change.[23]

Jiaogulan's ability to lower high blood pressure

General Summary

If the arterial blood pressure at the time of contraction (systole) of the heart exceeds 140mm Hg, and during expansion (diastole) is over 90mm Hg, then hypertension is diagnosed. Hypertension will cause serious complications of the brain, heart and kidneys. In China, physicians use gypenosides as a supplement for treatment of hypertension. On the other extreme, if systolic blood pressure is lower than 80mm Hg, and diastolic pressure lower than 60mm Hg, then hypotension is diagnosed. Hypotension will cause such bad effects as cerebral ischemia, collapse etc. Gypenosides are similar to the ginsenosides of Panax ginseng, in that they lower hypertension and raise hypotension, keeping the blood pressure at a normal range. The following study is a demonstration of jiaogulan's ability to lower high blood pressure.

Research

Laboratory experiments: A 1999 Vanderbilt University Medical Center study demonstrated that jiaogulan stimulates the release of nitric oxide, a substance that causes blood vessels in the body to relax. They concluded that this may be one mechanism by which jiaogulan reduces blood pressure.[23A]

Clinical Testing: Lu et al. studied the anti-hypertension effect of gypenosides in a double blind study. In this study, 223 patients with essential hypertension (Grade II) were randomly divided into 3 groups: Group 1 consisted of 76 patients; 20mg gypenosides tablets were administered orally, twice a day for three months. Group 2 consisted of 82 patients; 20mg ginsenosides tablets were administered orally, twice a day for 3 months. Group 3, 65 patients; 1.25mg Indapamide (an effective anti-hypertensive medicine, an alpha receptor inhibitor) was given orally, twice a day for three months. The results showed that the effectiveness rates were 82%, 46% and 93% for gypenosides, ginseng and Indapamide respectively.[24]

Jiaogulan's ability to lower cholesterol

General Summary

Jiaogulan has been shown to reduce the serum level of triglycerides, lipid peroxide, total cholesterol, phospholipids, and glutamic pyruvic transaminase in animal studies. These conditions are risk factors leading to hyperlipaemia, liver injury, and atherosclerosis. A great many human tests have confirmed jiaogulan's ability to lower serum cholesterol, triglycerides and LDL (unhealthy blood lipoprotein), while increasing HDL (healthy blood lipoprotein which helps to metabolize cholesterol from the arteries), thus preventing and treating atherosclerosis, heart attack and stroke.

Research

Animal Studies: Kimura et al. of Ehime University in Japan reported that crude saponins isolated from *Gynostemma pentaphyllum* were tested for their effect on lipid metabolism in rats which were fed a corn oil and high sugar diet. The oral administration of such high sugar and fat diet caused hyperlipaemia, liver injury with increased serum level of glutamic pyruvic transaminase, and accumulation of lipid peroxide in the liver. Administration of the crude saponins reduced serum levels of triglycerides, lipid peroxide, total cholesterol, phospholipids and glutamic pyruvic transaminase.[25]

Clinical Testing: Yu et al. of Hunan College of Traditional Chinese medicine carried out testing in 30 human cases with hyperproteinemia; the total effectiveness rate of jiaogulan to lower the high blood lipoprotein was 86.7%.[26]

Many clinical studies on the therapeutic effectiveness of jiaogulan/gypenosides on hyperlipemia have been reported in Chinese literature. Over 20 papers were published showing an effectiveness rate ranging between 67-93% on more than 980 patients with hyperlipemia. Most of the studies showed that jiaogulan/gypenosides lowered serum cholesterol, triglycerides, and LDL, while increasing HDL, thus decreasing the LDL/HDL ratio. Blood lipids include cholesterol and its ester, neutral fat (triglycerides) and phospholipids. They are not in free form but combine into various apolipoproteins, forming four types of water soluble lipoproteins: the chylomicron, very low density lipoprotein (VLDL), low density lipoprotein (LDL) and high density lipoprotein (HDL). VLDL, which is rich in triglycerides and LDL, which is rich in cholesterol ester, is closely related to the occurrence of atherosclerosis; whereas HDL, which acts as the carrier for cholesterol from the peripheral tissues to the liver and protects the endothelial cells from LDL damage, plays an important role against athero-sclerosis. A rise in blood lipoprotein (mainly LDL and VLDL-hyperlipoproteinemia), that is, a rise in blood lipids (mainly cholesterol and triglycerides-hyperlipemia) is the basis for occurrence of athero-sclerosis. Jiaogulan has been proven to affect the lipid metabolism by lowering the hyperproteinemia (name-ly hyperlipemia), thus preventing and treating athero-sclerosis.

Jiaogulan's ability to prevent heart attack and stroke

General Summary

The following tests show jiaogulan's ability to inhibit the aggregation of blood platelets. Platelet aggregation is the basis for formation of blood clots in the blood vessels of living ani-mals or humans (thrombosis) and accumulation of plaque in the arteries (atherosclerosis). Hence, the result of these tests suggest jiaogulan's ability to assist in preventing cerebral thrombosis, which results in stroke, and preventing coronary thrombosis, which results in acute heart attack.

Research

Laboratory Testing and Animal Studies: Tan et al. of the Guangzhou Medical College observed the anti-thrombotic effect of water extract of *Gynostemma pentaphyllum* both *in vitro* and *in vivo*, and found that it could inhibit significantly the platelet aggrega-tion induced by ADP and compound antagonists, accelerate obviously the dis-aggregation, and inhibit effectively the experimental thrombosis. The delaying effects of *Gynostemma pentaphyllum* on KPTT, PT,

TT, AT, RVV-RT, RVV-CT suggests that this herb could decrease the activity of multiple coagulation.[27]

Animal Study: Wu et al. showed that gypenosides inhibited rabbits' platelet aggregation induced by ADP through raising cAMP in the platelet and inhibiting the release of active factors from the platelet. They also reported that gypenosides could prevent thrombus formation in rats and inhibit the release of the thrombosis-related substances, 6-keto-PGF1a from the aorta and TXB2 from the platelet.[28]

Clinical Testing: Yu et al. performed a test in 56 healthy persons and 44 patients with cardiovascular diseases. The results showed that a single dose water extract of jiaogulan (containing gypenosides 30mg/1ml), 1ml/kg of body weight orally, inhibited platelet aggregation and promoted platelet dis-aggregation, indicating the anti-thrombotic effect of jiaogulan.[29]

Jiaogulan's ability to strengthen resistance
(enhancing white blood cell formation)

General Summary

Recovering from various illnesses and disease requires the strong assistance of the white blood cells. Jiaogulan affects the hematopoetic process, or the blood production process. Research has shown that it can increase the white blood cell count in leucopenic (white cell deficient) patients. Both of the following human tests confirm jiaogulan's ability to increase the white blood cell count of patients who were receiving both chemotherapy and radiation therapy, thus improving a patients ability to recover.

Research

Clinical Testing: Wang et al. treated 30 leucopenic patients with gypenosides and got marked effectiveness. The white blood count (WBC) of the peripheral blood before using gypenosides was 2.4 - 3.5 X 109 / L; after oral administration of gypenosides tablets (20mg) three times a day for one month, the WBC raised to 5.4 - 6.2 X 109 / L (P < 0.001).[30] Liu et al. used gypenosides to treat 90 cancer patients with leucopenia due to chemo-and/or radiotherapy and found marked effectiveness. They divided the patients into 3 groups: Group 1, 31 patients, were treated with jiaogulan and a traditional Chinese herb compound to treat leukopenia; Group 2, 31 patients, were treated with leukopoetic herb compound only; Group 3, the control group , 28 patients, were treated with a traditional Chinese health tonic. The overall WBC before using the recipes was 1.7 X 109 /L. In Group 1, the time it took the WBC to increase to over 4 X 109 /L averaged 4.69 days; the total effectiveness rate was 93.55%. In Group 2, the time it took the WBC count to rise above 4 X 109 /L averaged 7.22 days; the total effectiveness rate was 70.97%. In Group 3, the time it took the WBC to increase to over 4 X 109 /L averaged 22.82 days; the total effectiveness rate was 57.14%. (P <0,05, all the data compared with the data before treatment; the data of Group 1 compared with the respective data of Group 2. P < 0.01, the data of Group 1 compared with the respective data of Group 3).[31]

Strengthening immunity

General Summary

The following laboratory experiment and animal studies indicate that jiaogulan can enhance the immunity of immuno-deficient organisms (due to irradiation), as well as that of a normal, healthy organism. The mechanism by which jiaogulan acts is through modulating lymphocyte transformation and enhancing lymphocyte activity, since the lymphocyte activity and function are responsible for immunity of the organism. These tests suggest that jiaogulan can be used as an immunity enhancer for treatment of patients with immuno-deficiency due to irradiation, chemotherapy, and other causes. Human testing confirmed that jiaogulan/gypenosides enhance the cellular immunity (protective activity by lymphocytes) and humorous immunity (protection by antibody formation) of cancer patients whose immune function is lowered due to radiation or chemotherapy as well as due to the cancer growth itself.

Research

Laboratory Experiment: Liao et al. of Hengyang Medical College studied the effects of gypenosides on mouse splenic lymphocyte transformation and DNA polymerase ll activity in vitro, and found that gypenosides, 2.5-20mg/L enhanced splenic T- and B-cell transformation, increased the DNA synthesis, and potentiated the activity of DNA polymerase ll. This suggested that gypenosides regulated lymphocyte transformation and DNA synthesis by regulating DNA polymerase ll activity.[32]

Animal Study: Chen et al. of the Institute of Radiation Biology, National Tsing-Hua University in Taiwan studied the effects of gypenosides on cellular immunity of gamma ray irradiated mice and found that gypenosides were effective to enhance the recovery of body weight, splenic weight and immunocompetence in gamma ray irradiated mice from radiation damage.[33]

Clinical Testing: Hou et al. of the Academy of Medical Science of Hebei Province studied the effects of jiaogulan on the immunological function of cancer patients. Forty patients with various cancers were randomly divided into three groups after operations, chemo- and radiotherapy. For a period of three weeks, 13 patients were treated with 30 g per day of jiaogulan decocted in water; 11 cases were treated with jiaogulan plus small amounts of *Pericarpium Citri Reticulatae (chenpi), Fructus Crataegi (shanzha), Massa Fermentata Medicinalis (shenqu)* and *Endothelium Corneum (jineijin)*; and 16 cases treated with 30g of *Radix Astragali seu Hedysari (huangqi)*, also known as Astragalus, another adaptogenic herb, with the same additional ingredients as for the second group. Examination found that the LTT and IgG levels were significantly lower in the cancer patients than in the healthy subjects. The LTT level was significantly enhanced in the jiaogulan-treated group, which was quite similar to the results in the group treated with *Radix Astragali seu Hedysari*, well-known as an effective immuno-potentiator. The increase of LTT when chemotherapy was combined with the jiaogulan treatment suggested that the latter might possess a prophylactic effect for immunosuppression of chemotherapy.[34] Qian et al. of Shanghai Medical University studied the protective effect of jiaogulan on cellular immunity of patients with primary lung cancer treated by radiotherapy plus chemotherapy. One group received 80mg three times per day of jiaogulan tablets, the other group was the control. They found that jiaogulan could help the patients to maintain their cellular immunity as compared with the control group patients whose cellular immunity was further suppressed by radiation and chemotherapy, during the therapy period of sixty days. Comparing the jiaogulan group with the control group after a year, a trend appeared, showing that the prognosis of the jiaogulan-treated patients was superior to the control patients in terms of the medial time of distant metastasis, local tumor control rate and length of survival time. This study showed that jiaogulan could protect patients' cellular immunity when the patients were receiving radiation and chemotherapy.[35]

Jiaogulan's ability to inhibit the growth of cancer

General Summary

Ginsenoside Rh2 from ginseng is known to be effective in combating cancer cells. But only a very small amount of this type of saponin (0.001%) can be extracted from ginseng. The similar saponins, gypenosides 22-29 extracted from jiaogulan (also being more abundant than in ginseng) have been shown to be effective in controlling various types of cancer cells.[36,37] The following laboratory experiment shows the direct inhibitory effect of gypenosides from jiaogulan on tumor cells, indicating possible inhibitory effects in a living body. Animal tests have confirmed that jiaogulan can inhibit or prevent the malignant growth which was induced by introduction of a carcinogen. However, the effect of jiaogulan on cancer is still in the experimental stage up to date and its effect on human cancer needs further testing.

Research

Laboratory Experiment: Using the flow cytometry method, Han et al. of Shanghai University of Traditional Chinese medicine studied twenty-four Chinese medicinal herbs in a compound recipe on proliferation index, DNA index, protein index, and ratio of various phases in the cell cycle of the human lung adenocarcinoma cell. They found that Chinese medicinal herbs, such as jiaogulan, *Glehnia littoralis (beishashen)* and *Panax ginseng*, could strengthen the body resistance. They are not only useful as conventional tonics, but also as tumor cell inhibitors.[38]

Animal Study: Wang et al. of West China University of Medical Sciences performed an experiment on rats. The animals were given a 2% *Gynostemma pentaphyllum* boiled aqueous solution to drink freely for two weeks before administration of a carcinogen. Subsequently, the rats were injected with the carcinogen (MANA) for eighteen weeks and were sacrificed at intervals. The results showed that the number of tumors and the incidence of esophageal cancer in the experimental group were lower than those in the control group (MANA only), and the initiation of cancer was delayed for six weeks. This indicated that *Gynostemma pentaphyllum* might have some preventive and blocking effect on esophageal cancer in rats.[39]

Clinical Testing: Wu et al. reported that the effect of gypenosides enhanced the NK cell activity in patients with uro-genital cancers.[40]

Other therapeutic qualities of jiaogulan

Diabetes mellitus

General Summary

The following tests, both in animals and humans suggest that jiaogulan or its gypenosides might be used to treat diabetes mellitus. However, further studies are needed to confirm this effect.

Research

Animal Study: Cheng et al. used gypenosides to treat rats with diabetes mellitus for four weeks and found that the blood glucose, insulin, triglycerides, total cholesterol and MDA lowered markedly, while SOD increased.[41]

Clinical Testing: Cheng et al. used gypenosides to treat forty-six patients with diabetes mellitus for eight weeks. The results showed that the raised blood glucose, glycohemoglobin, cholesterol, triglycerides, LDL and blood viscosity were lowered to the normal range, whereas serum HDL increased. The percentage of the patients whose condition improved was 89.1%.[42] Wu et al. used gypenosides to treat 80 patients with type 2 diabetes mellitus and also got satisfactory results.[43]

Liver disorders

General Summary

Jiaogulan/gypenosides have been shown to be effective in treating liver damage and hepatitis.

Research

Laboratory Experiment: Hu et al. showed that gypenosides could protect cultured rats' liver cells from direct damage by carbon tetrachloride, a chemical compound exerting a toxic effect on the liver.[44]

Animal Study: Ye et al. and Du et al. consecutively reported protective effects of gypenosides on liver damage induced by carbon tetrachloride in rats.[45,46]

Clinical Testing: Zhu et al. used gypenosides to treat 100 patients with chronic hepatitis B for 3 months, and obtained satisfactory results, the effectiveness rate being 89%.[47] Ma et al. also treated 200 hepatitis B patients with gypenosides and saw a similar effect.[48]

Bronchitis

General Summary

One of the main traditional uses for which jiaogulan has been known was as a chronic bronchitis remedy. The following human test demonstrates its effectiveness.

Research

Liu et al. reported that in 86 cases of chronic bronchitis, the effectiveness rate of jiaogulan tea was 93%.[49] Hu et al. reported a 92% effectiveness rate in 96 cases of chronic bronchitis.[50]

Conclusion

As can be seen from the above results of extensive laboratory, animal and human research (50 studies have been cited here), jiaogulan has been shown to have many beneficial, preventive, and therapeutic effects on humans. These benefits have resulted in its extensive use as a therapeutic medicine in many hospitals throughout China. It seems timely now for researchers, natural health practitioners, and the health industry in general to look more seriously at the use of jiaogulan and jiaogulan based products as a beneficial addition to their range of health care supplements.

End Notes

1. Ma, Y.L., et al. Therapeutic effect of jiaogulan in 200 cases of hepatitis B. *Hebei Zhong XiYi Jie He Zazhi (Hebei Journal of combined Chinese and Western Medicine).* Chinese. 1997; 6(1): 48.
2. Cheng, H.W., et al. Clinical study on the effect of gypenosides on hyperlipaemia in 46 patients with diabetes mellitus. *Shiyong Zhong Xiyi Jiehe Zazhi (Journal of Applied Combined Chinese and Western Medicine).* Chinese, 1997; 10(19): 1879.
3. Xu, Shimin; Yao, Li; Wang, Yuanqing. Preparation of Gulanpenisong capsules and tablets containing *Gynostemma pentaphyllum* saponin and prednisone. *Faming Zhuanli Shenqing Gongkai Shuomingshu CN 1,088,783* (Cl. A61K31/70), July 6, 1994.
4. Xu, Shimin; Yao, Li; Wang, Yuanqing. Pharmaceutical tablets containing dexamethasone and *Gynostemma pentaphyllum* saponins. *Faming Zhuanli Shenqing Gongkai Shuomingshu CN 1,089,139* (Cl. A61K31/57), July 13, 1994.
5. Jin, M., et al. Effect of jiaogulan extract on a cell line from human rectal adenocarcinoma. *Xian Dai Yin Yong Yao Xue.* Chinese. 1992; 9(2): 49.
6. Li, G.Y. Effect of gypenosides on synthesis of DNA and protein of liver carcinoma cells in vitro. *Xian Yi Ke Da Xue Xue Bao.* Chinese. 1993; 14(2): 14.
7. Li, H. Inhibitory effect of gypenosides on lung cancer cells in vitro. *Xi An Yi Ke Da Xue Xue Bao.* Chinese. 1994; 15(4): 346.
8. Yang, Guiping, et al. Acute and long-term toxicological studies on gypenosides-containing tonics. *Guiyang Yixue Yuan Xuebao (Journal of Guiyang Medical College)* 1993 18(4):264.
9. Ibid.

10. Li, Lin, et al. Protective Effect of Gypenosides Against Oxidative Stress in Phagocytes, Vascular Endothelial Cells and Liver Microsomes. Loma Linda University, Calif. *Cancer Biotherapy* 1993; 8(3): 263-272.

11. Ibid.

12. Dai, D.Y., et al. The effect of antioxidant Chinese herbs on SOD activity, MDA content and ultrastructural damage of the brain tissue in mice with chronic fluorosis. *Zhongguo Di Fan Bing Zazhi (Chinese Journal of Endemic Diseases)*. Chinese. 1998; 17(4): 226.

13. Cheng, Y.H., et al. The effect of antioxidant Chinese herbs on SOD activity, MDA content and ultrastructural damage of the kidney tissue in mice with chronic fluorosis. *Guizhou Yiyao (Guizhou Medical Journal)*. Chinese.1998; 22(2): 94.

14. Lu, G.H., et al. The effect of antioxidant herbs on the erythrocytic SOD activity and serum MDA content in patients with endemic fluorosis. *Guizhou Medical Journal*. Chinese. 1998; 22(3): 25.

15. Liu, Jialiu, et al. Effects of a gypenosides-containing tonic on the serum SOD activity and MDA content in middle-aged and aged persons. *Journal of Guiyang Medical College* 1994; 19(1):17.

16. Zhang, X.L., et al. Study of the antioxidant effect of Danshen extract in aged persons and patients with fluorosis. *Zhonguo Di Fang Bing Zazhi (Chinese Journal of Endemic Diseases)*. Chinese. 1998; 17(4):234.

17. Zhou, S.R. A preliminary study on the effects of *Gynostemma pentaphyllum* on endurance, spontaneous motor activity and superoxide dismutase in mice. *Asia Pacific Journal of Pharmacology* 1990; 5(4): 321-322.

18. Song, W.M., et al. Comparison of the adaptogenic effect of jiaogulan and ginseng. *Zhong Cao Yao*. Chinese. 1992; 23(3): 136.

19. Zhang, Yi-Qun, et al. Immediate effects of a gypenosides-containing tonic on the echocardiography of healthy persons of various ages. *Journal of Guiyang Medical College* 1993; 18(4):261.

20. Zhou, Ying-Na, et al. Influence of kiwifruit/jiaogulan recipe on the lung function and exercise endurance under exercise workload. *Journal of Guiyang Medical College*. Chinese. 1993; 18(4): 256.

21. Liu, Jialiu, et al. Overall health-strengthening effects of a gypenosides-containing tonic in middle-aged and aged persons. *Journal of Guiyang Medical College*. 1993; 18(3):146.

22. Chen, L.F., et al. Comparison between the effects of gypenosides and ginsenosides on cardiac function and hemodynamics in dogs. *Zhongguo Yaolixue Yu Dulixue Zazhi*. Chinese. 1990; 4(1): 17-20.

23. Zhou, Ying-Na, et al. Effects of a gypenosides-containing tonic on the pulmonary function in exercise workload. *Journal of Guiyang Medical College* 1993 18(4):261.

23A. Tanner, M.A., et al. The direct release of nitric oxide by gypenosides derived from the herb Gynostemma pentaphyllum. Nitric Oxide 1999 Oct;3(5):359-65.

24. Lu, G.H., et al. Comparative study on anti-hypertensive effect of Gypenosides, Ginseng and Indapamide in patients with essential hypertension. *Guizhou Medical Journal.* Chinese. 1996; 20:1.

25. Kimura, Y., et al. Effects of crude saponins of Gynostemma pentaphyllum on lipid metabolism. *Shoyakugaku Zasshi.* Japanese. 1983 (Rec'd 1984); 37(3): 272-275.

26. Yu, C. Therapeutic effect of Tablet gypenosides on 32 patients with hyperlipaemia. *Hu Bei Zhong Yi Za Zhi.* Chinese. 1993; 15(3): 21.

27. Tan, H., et al. Antithrombotic effect of *Gynostemma pentaphyllum. Chung Kuo Chung HsiI Chieh Ho Tsa Chih (BIF).* Chinese. 1993 May; 13(5): 278-280, 261.

28. Wu, Jiliang, et al. Effects of gypenosides on platelet aggregation and cAMP levels in rabbits. *Zhongguo Yaolixue Yu Dulixue Zazhi.* Chinese. 1990; 4(1): 54-57.

29. Yu, J., et al. The effect of jiaogulan on aggregation and dis-aggregation of human platelets. *Fujian Yixue Yuan Xuebao (Journal of Fujian Medical College).* Chinese. 1995; 29(3): 246.

30. Wang, H.R., et al. Therapeutic and tonic effects of jiaogulan on leukopenic patients. *Xin Zhong Yi.* Chinese. 1991; 23(1): 36.

31. Liu, et al. Therapeutic effect of jiaogulan on leukopenia due to irradiation and chemotherapy. *Zhong Guo yi Yao Xue Bao.* Chinese. 1992; 7(2): 99.

32. Liao, D.F., et al. Effects of gypenosides on mouse splenic lymphocte transformation and DNA polymerase II activity in vitro. *Acta Pharmacologica Sinica.* 1995; 16(4): 322-324.

33. Chen, W.C., et al. Protective effects of Gynostemma pentaphyllum on cellular immunity of gamma-ray-irradiated mice. *American Journal of Chinese Medicine* 1996; 24(1): 83.

34. Hou, J., et al. Effects of Gynostemma pentaphyllum makino on the immunological function of cancer patients. *Journal of Traditional Chinese Medicine (K9K)* 1991; 11(1): 47-52.

35. Qian, Hao, et al. Protective effect of jiaogulan on cellular immunity of the patients with primary lung cancer treated by radiotherapy plus chemotherapy. *Acta Academiae Medicinae Shanghai* 1995; 22(5): 363-366.

36. Takemoto, T., et al. *Health Before You Know It. Amachazuru.* Yutaka Nakano Shobo; 1984; p. 36.

37. Zhou, He-Ping. The saponin constituents and pharmacology of Gynostemma pentaphyllum Makino. *Yaoxue Tongbao.* Chinese. 1988; 23(12): 720-724.

38. Han, M.Q., et al. Effects of 24 Chinese medicinal herbs on nucleic acid, protein and cell cycle of human lung adenocarcinoma cell. *Chung Kuo Chung His I Chieh Ho Tsa Chih (BIF).* Chinese. 1995 Mar; 15(3): 147-9.

39. Wang, Chao-Jun, et al. A preliminary observation of preventive and blocking effect of Gynostemma pentaphyllum (Thunb.) Makino on esophageal cancer in rats. *Huaxi Yixue Yuan Xuebao (Journal of West China University of Medical Sciences).* Chinese. 1995; 26(4): 430-432.

40. Wu, J.L., et al. Influence of gypenosides on thrombosis and synthesis of TXA2 and PGF1a. *Zhong Yao Yao Li Yu Lin Chuang.* Chinese. 1991; 7(2): 39.

41. Cheng, H.W., et al. The effect of gypenosides to lower the hyperglycemia in rats with diabetes mellitus. *Chinese Journal of Diabetes Mellitus.* Chinese. 1997; 5(4): 229.

42. Cheng, H.W., et al. Clinical study on the effect of gypenosides on hyperlipaemia in 46 patients with diabetes mellitus. *Shiyong Zhong Xiyi Jiehe Zazhi* (Journal of Applied Combined Chinese and Western Medicine). Chinese. 1997; 10(19): 1879.

43. Wu, P.K., et al. Therapeutic effect of a compound jiaogulan recipe to treat 80 patients with type ll diabetes mellitus. *Hunan Journal of Chinese Medicine.* Chinese. 1997; 13(6): 7.

44. Hu, B.C., et al. The protective effect of gypenosides on the cultured rat's liver cells against direct damage by carbon tetrachloride. *Hengyang Yixue Yuan Xuebao (Journal of Hengyang Medical College).* Chinese. 1996; 24(4): 268.

45. Ye, Z.J., et al. The effect of jiaogulan to reduce lipid peroxidation of rat liver caused by carbon tetrachloride. *Gong Yewei Sheng Yuzi Yebing (Industrial Hygeine and Professional Diseases).* Chinese. 1998; 24(2): 74.

46. Du, Y.Y., et al. Protective effect of gypenosides and organic Ge compound on the liver against carbon tetrachloride damage. *Ziye Yixue (Professional Medicine).* Chinese 1996; 23(3): 46.

47. Zhu, B.Z. Therapeutic effect of jiaogulan granules on 100 patients with chronic hepatitis B. *Anhui Zhong Yixue Yuan Xue Bao (Journal of Anhui College of Traditional Chinese Medicine).* Chinese. 1994; 13(3): 7.

48. Ma, Y.L., et al. Therapeutic effect of jiaogulan in 200 cases of hepatitis B. *Hebei Zhong XiYi Jie He Zazhi (Hebei Journal of combined Chinese and Western Medicine)*. Chinese. 1997; 6(1): 48.

49. Liu, Z.X. Therapeutic effect of jiaogulan on 86 patients with chronic bronchitis. *Hunan Zhong Yi Za Zhi. (Hunan Journal of Traditional Chinese Medicine)*. Chinese. 1993; 9(4): 11.

50. Hu, B.C., et al. Therapeutic effect of gypenosides in 96 cases of chronic bronchitis. *Zhong Cao Yao Yan Jiu (Research on Chinese Herbs)*. Chinese. 1996; 4, 136.

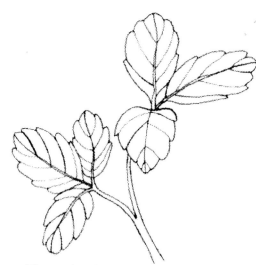

Three-leaf jiaogulan

Chapter Four

Botany and Culti-vation

Jiaogulan is a plant of the genus *Gynostemma*. It belongs to the family Cucurbitaceae (cucumber or gourd, which includes melons), how-

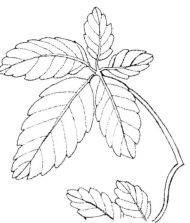

Five-leaf jiaogulan

ever without the characteristic fruit.[1]

There are over thirty species of *Gynostemma* growing throughout China, with many of them growing abundantly in the Southwest. Most

Seven-leaf jiaogulan

of the species have other Asian distribution in at least one or two countries. The *pentaphyllum* species, however, is the most widespread, with distribution in Bangladesh, India, Japan, Korea, Laos, Myanmar, Nepal, Sri Lanka and Vietnam.[2] The botanical names of some of the species are listed below.

Gynostemma aggregatum C.Y. Wu & S.K. Chen, 1983

Gynostemma burmanicum King ex Chakr., 1946

Gynostemma burmanicum var. *burmanicum*

Gynostemma burmanicum var. *molle* C.Y. Wu in C.Y. Wu & S.K. Chen, 1983

Gynostemma cardiospermum Cogn. Ex Oliv. In Hook. F., 1894

Gynostemma compressum XX Chen & D.R. Liang, 1991

Gynostemma guangxiense X.X. Chen & D.H. Qin, 1988

Gynostemma laxiflorum C.Y. Wu & S.K. Chen, 1983

Gynostemma laxum (Wall.) Cogn. In A. DC., 1881

Gynostemma longipes C.Y. Wu in C.Y. Wu & S.K. Chen, 1983

Gynostemma microspermum C.Y. Wu & S.K. Chen, 1983

Gynostemma pallidinerve Z. Zhang, 1991

Gynostemma pentagynum Z.P. Wang, 1989

Gynostemma pentaphyllum (Thunb.) Makino, 1902

Gynostemma pentaphyllum var. dasycarpum C.Y. Wu & C.Y. Wu & S.K. Chen, 1983

Gynostemma pentaphyllum var. *pentaphyllum*

Gynostemma pubescens (Gagnep. In Lecomte) C.Y. Wu in C.Y. Wu & S.K. Chen, 1983

Gynostemma simplicifolium Blume, 1825

All of the above species are called "jiaogulan" in Chinese. The species other than *Gynostemma pentaphyllum* (Thunb.) Makino have various modifying Chinese words before "jiaogulan". "Jiaogulan" without a modifying word usually indicates *Gynostemma pentaphyllum* (Thunb.) Makino. Most of the sci-

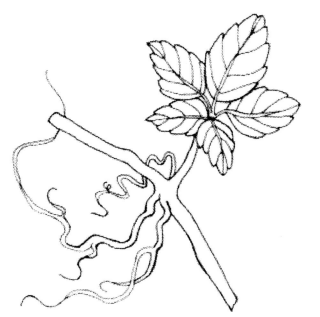

Root cutting with leaf

entific studies have been performed using this species. However, many of the species of the genus *Gynostemma* have been used as a medicinal herb in China, all containing similar effective components and exerting similar functions.

In China, one or more of the above jiaogulan species can be found growing wild in the provinces of Shaanxi, Sichuan, Yunnan, Guizhou, Guangxi, Hubei, Hunan, Jiangsu,

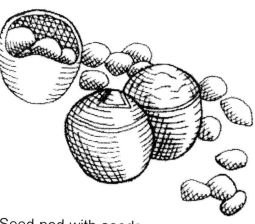

Seed pod with seeds

Zhejiang, Anhui, and Hainan. Jiaogulan can be found growing in the mountains and plains, at an elevational range of between 1,000 and 10,000 feet (300-3200 meters).[3]

Jiaogulan is an easily grown herbaceous perennial vine, which requires a rich well drained humus rich soil in a warm sheltered area with partial shade. It does not grow well in cold climates where temperatures drop down to freezing. It can be grown successfully year round in a greenhouse, or indoors but requires warm (but not too dry) weather if it is to do well out-doors. A climbing plant, attaching itself to supports by means of tendrils, Jiaogulan is dioecious, meaning male and female plants must be grown to produce fertile seeds.

Jiaogulan: China's "Immortality" Herb

Dr. Takemoto, in his book on amachazuru (jiaogulan), describes the physical characteristics of the herb in detail, as follows: "Amachazuru is a vine weed, similar in appearance to sorrel vine (of the grape family), Japanese hop (mulberry fam-

Dammarane framework
of jiaogulan and ginseng

Testosterone

Bile acid

ily), and joe pye weed (eggplant family). It has subterranean shoots (rootstocks) and its stems grow like vines. A thick, curled hair grows near the root of the leaf stem which has alternatively growing leaves, either of three, five or seven. The plant has male and female roots. The leaf is oval-shaped with sawtooth edges, on which grow fine, white hairs. In the summer the plant gives blossom to pale yellow flowers. The female plant bears berries which turn black when ripe and contain its seeds. Jiaogulan can be cultivated from the seed or from plant cuttings."[4]

To cultivate by seed: Pre-soak seeds for about 2 days in warm water before planting. To cultivate by plant cuttings: Cover the growing vine with earth. When it takes root in about 20 days, make a cutting by slicing off the rooted section on either side of the roots, then plant in rich soil. Fertilize around the root, not directly at the roots.

Like most perennial plants, the rate of growth increases as the plant establishes a more extensive root system. Jiaogulan is a fast-growing plant, as much as 2.5 inches overnight. A new plant may be expected to produce several stems which will grow 3'-6' in the first year (depending on climate and length of growing season in your area). The plant is killed to the ground by a freeze, but will begin growth again in late spring. In cold areas it is advisable to protect the roots with a good layer of mulch during the winter. Jiaogulan tends to grow very profusely in the wild. However, since jiaogulan has been recognized as an important medicinal herb, artificial cultivation has been researched in China, Korea, and Japan. The following are some studies that have been made to seek out the best methods of cultivation, crop management, and harvesting for large scale agronomic production.

In China, Zhou et al. studied the gypenoside concentration of jiaogulan harvested in various seasons and reported that in artificial cultivation jiaogulan harvested in June (early summer season) contained the highest gypenoside concentration. As for wild-growing plants, August (late summer season) was the best harvest time, when jiaogulan contained the highest gypenoside concentration.[5] Xiao et al. conducted studies on semi-culture techniques, intercropping techniques, agronomic standardization, and a development model for large scale production of jiaogulan.[6] Huang et al. recommended a new method of cultivation with cutting leaves. They reported that this method could be used for developing jiaogulan of a high quality in a large growing area.[7] In Korea, Seong et al. confirmed that the leaf-cutting culture methods (mentioned in the previous study) were best for good rooting of "Dungkulcha" (Korean name for jiaogulan).[8]

End Notes

1. Flora of China Study. Missouri Botanical Garden. *www.mobot.org* June 1998.
2. Ibid.
3. Ibid.
4. Takemoto, Tsunematsu., et al., *Health Before You Know It. Amachazuru.* Eng. Yutaka Nakano Shobo 1984.
5. Zhu, S.X., et al. Detection of gypenoside concentration in jiaogulan harvested at different times. *Hunan Zhongyi Zazhi.* Chinese. 1990; 6(4): 52.
6. Xiao, X.H., et al. Distribution and resources of Genus *Gynostemma* in Shichuan. *Zhong Yao Cai.* Chinese. 1991; 14(3): 16.
7. Huang, T.F. New techniques for heightening the production quantity of jiaogulan in cultivation. *Zhong Cao Yao.* Chinese. 1993; 24(12): 648.
8. Seong, J.D., et al. Characteristics, distribution and propagation methods of medicinal crop Dungkulcha, *Gynostemma pentaphyllum. Res. Rep. Rural Dev. Adm (Suweon) 31(3 Upland Ind. Crops)* Philippine. 1989; 57-61.

Chapter Five

Chemical Components of Jiaogulan

Jiaogulan contains saponins, flavones, polysaccharides, amino acids, vitamins, and minerals, including many essential trace elements. Among these, the saponins are the most important of the effective components.

What exactly is a saponin? A saponin is a high-molecular-weight glycoside, consisting of two components: the aglycone and, attached to it, a sugar molecule. Saponins have the unique quality of dissolving in both water and oil, and when mixed with water and shaken, it will foam up. The particular type of saponins of both jiaogulan (gypenosides) and *Panax ginseng* (ginsenosides) are classified as belonging to the dammarane diol family, containing a dammarane framework as their basic chemical structure, hence both herbs exert similar effects on the human body. This dammarane structure is similar to the chemical structure of steroid hormones, a group of compounds occurring naturally in the bodies of animals and humans, and which play important roles in regulating a number of bodily systems.[1] However, these steroid-like components do not have a direct hormonal action, but only influence the body to produce a healthy balance (homoestasis) of hormones. (It should be noted here, for the benefit of athletes, that the steroid-like dammarane structures of jiaogulan and ginseng can be detected *without* being confused with steroid hormones, such as androgen, testosterone, or corticosterone. In other words, neither jiaogulan nor ginseng are banned substances by the International Olympic Committee.) Note the similarity between the chemical structure of gypenosides and our body's own steroids. This similarity might contain the secret of its energizing, balancing, and therapeutic effects.[2] The saponins are the effective components that account for the health benefits explained in detail in Chapter 3. The eighty-two saponins of jiaogulan have been given the nomenclature "gypenosides," which scientists assigned to it because of the botanical name, *Gynostemma pentaphyllum*. They took the first few letters from both the genus and specie, that is, *Gy* and *pen*, and added to it the suffix *-oside*, which refers to the saponins, hence gypenosides. The saponins of *Panax ginseng* were named in a similar way, therefore they are known as either *panax*-osides or *ginsen*-osides.

Out of the eighty-two gypenosides of jiaogulan, four of them are exactly the same as four ginsenosides of ginseng, in chemical structure and function. Gypenoside #'s 3, 4, 8, and 12 are exactly like ginsenoside Rb1, Rb3, Rd, and F2 respectively.[3] Seventeen other gypenosides, when hydrolyzed, have been found to be similar to those found in ginseng. Jiaogulan differs from that of *Panax ginseng* in that most herbalists offer a caution to persons with high blood pressure to avoid higher doses of *Panax ginseng*.[4] There are no such cautions with jiaogulan.

End Notes

1. Takemoto, Tsunematsu., et al. *Health Before You Know It. Amachazuru.* Eng. Yutaka Nakano Shobo 1984.
2. Ibid.
3. Takemoto, Tsunematsu, et al. Studies of the constituents of *Gynostemma pentaphyllum* Makino. I. Structures of Gypenosides I-XIV. *Yakugakuzasshi* 1983; 103(2): 173-185.
4. Hobbs, Christopher. *The Ginsengs* 1996; Botanica Press.

Chapter Six

Jiaogulan Products

Owing to its wide variety of therapeutic effectiveness, jiaogulan has been popularly used as a tonic and medicinal herb in China, and has more recently been introduced in the U.S. There are many different forms of jiaogulan products that have been developed. The traditional way that it has been used for many years is as a tea, but because of the great quantity of scientific testing, many of the products are now being made from the standardized gypenoside extract of jiaogulan, either as a single herb supplement or in combination with other Chinese herbs. Still other products are made using a concentrated extract.

Different growing conditions can affect the quantity of the effective components produced by a plant. Therefore, in order to properly evaluate the effects of an herb, scientists have "standardized" the active component-by isolating and measuring it. A complete isolation would be 100%, and in the case of jiaogulan would be called 100% gypenosides. An 85% gypenosides product would therefore contain 15% of other parts of the plant. Many traditional herbalists, however, feel that the whole raw herb, with its entire spectrum of components, is more

*Individual products with additional herbs combined with gypenosides, due to an enhanced synergistic effect, may not require as much gypenosides as recommended below. Consult an herbalist or the company itself for advice. Then again, some herbalists may recommend much larger doses than listed here, particularly for the more serious life-threatening diseases, since some of the studies confirm not only the usefulness but also the acceptability of higher doses.

effective than isolating and standardizing the main component, since it might exclude other vital ingredients during the extracting processes. This is a debate that has existed between traditional practitioners and medical researchers since the advent of the common availability of standardized ingredients.[1] There are arguments on both sides of the issue, however, until there are side-by-side comparative studies, the debate will not be concluded. What we do know in the case of jiaogulan is that a great deal of animal tests and clinical tests on humans have shown that the chief components, pure gypenosides, are extremely effective for use as a therapeutic and medicinal herb treatment. And yet traditional Chinese herbalists have been using non-standardized, full spectrum herbs for thousands of years.

In products not using the standardized extract of gypenosides, you might not know how much jiaogulan you are actually getting, or if the quality will be consistent. As is always the case, "buyer beware!" Try to buy from a company with a reputation for quality. However, at the time of this printing, it is not likely that any companies are selling what I call "decaf jiaogulan," that is, a jiaogulan extract with the active ingredient (the gypenosides) removed. The gypenosides that would be removed are then used in other forms, such as capsules or tablets. This is the practice of some unethical companies who sell very inexpensive, so-called ginseng, and thereby cheat the innocent public. The active ingredient, the ginsenosides, have been removed for use in other products and what remains is sold as ginseng. Well, you're getting ginseng, but without the effects of ginseng. The same thing could happen to jiaogulan, so be forewarned.

The following is a list of the various forms in which jiaogulan is available:

Jiaogulan Tea: Several kinds of tea are made and are popularly used in China. A tea is often used as a daily

71

tonic for long-term use. Chinese people have reported increase of vitality and endurance, relief from fatigue, improvement of appetite, improvement of sleep and enhanced resistance to disease as a result of using the tea. Teas are made of dried jiaogulan leaves, since the highest concentration of saponins is in the leaves; still, the entire plant (if available) could be chopped and used as a tea. Among the many species of jiaogulan there are not only differences in saponin content, but also a variation of tastes. They can be divided into sweet, slightly sweet, bitter and tasteless. Most of the species growing are bitter. However, there are some slightly sweet and sweet varieties available in the marketplace. Such teas are exported to the U.S., where *Gynostemma pentaphyllum* tea bags can be found at Chinese herb shops, health food stores, or ordered through many online companies. (See Appendix.)

Jiaogulan Wine: Studies in China showed that the alcoholic extract is as effective as the water extract from jiaogulan.[2] Jiaogulan wine has been produced and distributed by the Shandong Wine Factory and is very popular in China. At present, it is not sold in the U.S.

Jiaogulan Gel-caps or Capsules: These can contain jiaogulan in either standardized extract form or as a concentrated, non-standardized extract. If it contains a standardized extract, the label will usually say *standardized gypenosides*, with the amount in milligrams. If it is a non-standardized extract, it will simply say *Gynostemma pentaphyllum* or jiaogulan with the appropriate amount of milligrams, or you may inquire from the company. They can be found in the U.S in

Chinese herb shops and are available from some herb companies. (See Appendix)

Jiaogulan Tea-pills: These are round, ¼ inch diameter, brown-colored pills made from a 4:1 (approx.) concentrated jiaogulan tea. (See Appendix for availability.)

Gypenoside Tablet: One company that manufactures this product is Guangxi Health Tonic and Pharmaceutical Factory in China. Each tablet contains 10 mg of purified total gypenosides extracted from jiaogulan. It is used as a tonic for health support and nourishment, and also as a supplemental medicine for treating atherosclerosis, hypertension, cancer, and other diseases as mentioned previously. Its dosage is 1-2 tablets (10-20 mg) 3 times a day. These might be found at Chinese herb shops.

Gypenoside Liquid (Oral): This product is made of a water solution in which the powdered gypenosides have been mixed. It is produced by a few companies in China, the most popular being the Xi-Xiou Pharmaceutical Factory. It comes in 10 mg doses in 10 ml vials, ten vials to a box. The dosage and usage are the same as for the tablets. They might be sold in Chinese herb shops.

Gypenoside/Herb Combination: This is a product that contains other standardized ingredients having either similar or complementary qualities that act in synergy with standardized gypenosides to produce more powerful therapeutic effects. In one product manufactured by Jagulana Herbal Products, gypenosides are combined with the Chinese herb Danshen in a base of kiwi fruit. This can be found in natural products stores in the U.S. To give an idea of how the combination works, the resulting synergy is explained like this:

1) In terms of anti-oxidation, the gypenosides induce the synthesis of superoxide dismutase (SOD), which scavenges excessive free radicals The kiwi fruit is rich in vitamin C and E, which capture free radicals and reacts with them, thus breaking off their action on the cell membrane lipids. The Danshen clears out the free radicals and MDA, a toxic lipid-peroxidation product, and directly protects the cell membrane from injury by free radicals and MDA. These three act at various levels, exerting a synergistic effect, efficiently inhibiting the peroxidation of lipids in the membranous structure of the cells.

2) Regarding the synergistic effect on cardiovascular function, gypenosides enhance the cardiac contraction and stroke volume, increasing cardiac output into the blood vessels, without increasing the heart rate. Danshen improves the micro-circulation of musculature and viscera. These two herbs act at different levels; i.e., affecting the heart muscle itself as well as the peripheral vasculature or circulation, thus exerting an effect of improved efficiency of physical and athletic performance.

See Appendix for names and addresses of companies selling jiaogulan products.

Preventative and Therapeutic Suggestions

Based on the dosages used in medical research studies and those recommended on commercial products sold in China, we have compiled the following list of suggested dosages of 85% gypenosides for specific uses, both preventive and therapeutic.*

Antioxidant protection—20mg/3 times/day

Adaptogenic—20mg/3 times/day

Enhancing cardio-vascular function—20mg/2 or 3 times/day

General illness prevention (general health maintenance) — 20mg/2 or 3 times/day

Lowering high blood pressure
        preventive—20mg/2 or 3 times/day
        therapeutic—60mg/2 or 3 times/day

Lowering cholesterol
        preventive—20mg/2 or 3 times/day
        therapeutic—60mg/3 times/day

Inhibiting platelet aggregation (protection against heart attack and stroke)
        preventive—20mg/1 or 2 times /day
        therapeutic—60mg/3 times/day

Enhancing white blood cell formation
        preventive—20mg/2 or 3 times /day
        therapeutic (during radio-and chemotherapy and other conditions which might cause leukopenia)—60mg/3 times/day

Strengthening immunity (during various weakening situations; for example radio- and chemotherapy, and other illnesses)— 60mg/2 or 3 times /day

Cancer inhibition
        preventive—20mg/2 times/day
        therapeutic (as a supplementary therapy to radio- or chemotherapy or surgery)—60mg/ 3 times/day

Others—diabetes, liver disorders, bronchitis—20mg/ 3 times/day

End Notes

1. Hobbs, Christopher. Gingko, *Elixir of Youth*, 1991; Botanica Press, p. 58.
2. Qu, A.K., et al. Comparative study on the gypenosides content in alcoholic extract and water extract of jiaogulan. *Shi Pin Wei Sheng (Foods*

and Health) Chinese, 1993; p. 34.

Chapter Seven

Frequently Asked Questions

Q: *Is jiaogulan addicting?*
A: No. It is not addicting at all. Although it adjusts the function of the central nervous system, calming the brain when it is irritated, exciting it when it is depressed, it is neither a central nervous system stimulant nor a sedative.

Q: *Will it keep me awake at night?*
A: Since gypenosides exert a bi-phasic action on the central nervous system, jiaogulan will help you get to sleep easier, because it will calm the nerves and mental irritations by helping to balance the sympathetic and parasympathetic nerves. But if you want to work at night, take a bigger dose of jiaogulan (twice the ordinary dose); then it will keep you awake, and in good spirits, as well.

Q: *I'm a distance runner. What is jiaogulan going to do for me?*
A: Jiaogulan increases cardiac output and improves oxygen absorption, thereby delaying lactic acid production and fatigue; and as an antioxidant it speeds recovery. Besides, it increases the excitability and stability of the brain, hence making you more adapted to the intensity of competition, to heighten your performance.

Q: *Will jiaogulan speed up my heart rate?*

A: No. In fact, athletes who use a heart rate monitor have seen a lower heart rate, when taking jiaogulan during exercise (at the same workload) than without taking jiaogulan. Research has shown that after taking jiaogulan, cardiac output increased mainly through increase in stroke volume, not through increase in heart rate. This means that the heart contracts more powerfully, and hence works more efficiently.

Q: *How long do the effects last?*
A: During non-training, non-workout, or non-exercise, four hours. During medium intensity training, workout, or exercise, three hours. During events, high intensity training, workouts, or exercise, two hours.

Q: *How does it reduce cholesterol?*
A: The proposed mechanism of action of gypenosides is the same as many other saponin-based foods or herbs-that they act by binding with bile acids and cholesterol, thus making the molecule too big to be absorbed. In this way it is thought that saponins "clean" or purge these fatty compounds from the body, lowering the blood cholesterol levels.

Q: *How can it give me energy when I'm tired, yet relax me when I go to bed?*
A: When you are tired and your brain is depressed, jiaogulan first of all excites your brain, then excites the sympathetic nervous system, which in turn stimulates the secretions of the adrenal gland and thyroid gland. By jiaogulan's effect on neuro-endocrine adjustment, the metabolism increases, thus supplying you more energy. It calms down your nerves and mental irritation when you go to bed.

Q: *What effect does jiaogulan have on my blood pressure?*
A: It has a regulating effect, in that it helps to lower high blood pressure and raise low blood pressure. If your blood

pressure is within the normal range, it does not affect your blood pressure at all.

Q: *How can an herb (jiaogulan) relieve stress?*

A: As we have mentioned in Chapter 3, stress caused by various strong environmental and psychological stimuli creates stress syndrome by which the equilibrium of the central nervous system is disturbed. Then the central nervous system's normal regulation on the endocrine glands and various systems and organs is disturbed, and then equilibrium between various organs and the interior stability of the organism (homeostasis) is disturbed. Human and animal testing has proven jiaogulan/gypenosides to be a highly effective adaptogenic tonic. It exerts a bi-phasic action on the central nervous system, calming the nerves when they were irritated while exciting the nerves when they were depressed. Through adjusting the balance of the central nervous system (including the brain), the sympathetic and parasympathetic nervous systems, and toning the endocrine system, it maintains and normalizes the functional equilibrium between the organs and the stability of the organism, hence relieving stress.

Q: *What will jiaogulan do for my menstrual cramps?*

A: There is no information about the effect of jiaogulan on menstrual cramps. It has been noted that a tonic made of gypenosides in combination with Dong Quai and other herbs to treat menorrhagia has gotten good effects. In such case, jiaogulan, as an adaptogen, acts in synergism with Dong Quai, adjusting the activity of the genital tract directly and through the neuro-endocrine regulation as well.

Q: *I already take plenty of anti-oxidants; why should I take jiaogulan?*

A: Various anti-oxidants act at various levels and by different mechanisms. Jiaogulan induces the body's own production of SOD, a strong natural scavenger for free radicals, thus protecting the cells from free radical damage. It will also act in synergy with other anti-oxidants, increasing the anti-oxidation effect.

Q: *I have mitral valve prolapse. Will jiaogulan help?*
A: Jiaogulan can be helpful. Mitral valve prolapse occurs in middle-aged and aged persons, due to a degenerative change of the valve. It creates an overloading of the heart cells and causes mitral valve insufficiency in severe cases. Jiaogulan improves the nourishment and metabolism of the overloaded and weakened myocardium, thus benefiting the heart.

Q: *Is jiaogulan beneficial for menopause?*
A: Yes, it is. Jiaogulan calms the brain, balances the activity of central nervous system, the sympathetic and parasympathetic nervous systems, and adjusts the neuro-endocrine regulation of the genital system, thus relieving menopausal symptoms.

Q: *I'm sixty-five and suffering from impotence. Will jiaogulan improve my sexual ability?*
A: Jiaogulan may help in some forms of impotence because of jiaogulan's ability to improve circulation. Many men suffer from impotence because of impaired circulation.

Q: *I get pretty bad PMS each month. Will jiaogulan help?*
A: Jiaogulan acts by the mechanism similar to that in the case of menopausal syndrome; therefore, it tends to be beneficial to persons suffering from **PMS** symptoms.

Q: *Will jiaogulan do anything for my arthritis?*
A: There are a few studies reporting that jiaogulan improved the symptoms of arthritis.

Q: *Are there any side effects from taking jiaogulan?*
A: There are no known side effects at normal dosages. Side

Book Order Form

📠 Telephone Orders: Call 1-888-TORCHLT (1888-867-2458)
Have your Visa, Mastercard or American Express Card ready

📄 FAX Orders: (559) 337-2354

✉ Postal Orders: Torchlight Publishing
PO Box 52
Badger CA 93603

💻 Internet Orders: www.torchlight.com

Please send the following: QTY:

Jiaogulan: China's "Immortality " Herb $7.95 x _____ = $ _____
by Michael Blumert and Dr. Jialiu Liu

Sales tax: (CA residents add 7.25%) $ _____

Shipping and Handling (see below) $ _____

Total $ _____

O Please send me more information on other books published by
Torchlight Publishing

Company: _____

Name: _____

Address: _____

City: _____State_____Zip_____

(I understand I may return any books for a full refund, for any reason.)

O Check/Money Order enclosed   O VISA   O MasterCard   O American
Express

Card number: _____ Exp. Date:_____

Name on card: _____

Signature: _____

Shipping and Handling:
USA: $2.00 for first book; $1.00 each additional book.
Priority Mail (USA only): $3.20 per book.
Canada: $3.00 first book; $1.50 each additional book.
All Other Countries: $6.00 first book; $3.00 each additional book:
Allow 6 to 8 weeks for overseas delivery.